"I invite women to consider that our bellies
shelter creative energy
that's kin to the majestic Power of Being informing the universe."

"Our ancestors
considered a woman's belly to be sacred, not shameful.
Maybe our ancestors got it right."

Lisa Sarasohn
The Woman's Belly Book.

the MOON and YOU

A Woman's Guide to an Easier Monthly Cycle

Discover your own Inner Rhythms and Take Loving Care of Yourself

by Barbara Hanneloré
Author of
How to Celebrate Your Daughter's Coming of Age

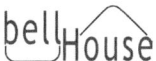

Copyright 2014 by Barbara Hanneloré

All rights reserved. No part of this book may be reproduced or utilized in any form or by any means, electronic or mechanical, including photocopying, recording, or by any information storage and retrieval system, without permission in writing from the publisher.

Printed and bound in the United States by Printing Impressions

ISBN 978-0-578-13156-6

Text design and layout by Cynthia Smith
Cover design and layout by Heather Wennergren and Barbara Hanneloré
Illustrations by Barbara Hanneloré

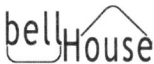

Bell House ☖ PO Box 1096 ☖ Goleta , CA, 93116

Praise
For Women's Way Moon Cycles

"When I first started talking to you, I had no idea about my cycle. I had no idea that the first days were connected to the last days…that ovulation had anything to do with my period. I didn't even realize my cycle was 29 days long, like the moon. All I knew was that I didn't want those three days when I bled. I didn't pay any attention to the rest. After learning more about it, all that changed and became so much better. I understood it."
~Renee H., realtor, Houston, TX

"I thought I was liberated because I ignored my cycle. Now, I see what I've been missing, and I want to pay attention…especially to the spiritual part."
~Jenna S., student, Ventura, CA

"Barbara, after your class I looked forward to my period! That was a first!"
~Gail M., teacher, Santa Barbara, CA

Praise for The Moon and You

"It's about time a book like this was written. It really validates and celebrates the sacredness of our bodies and cycles. If you're in tune with your cycle, the awareness is huge, profound. It expands your ability to be fully aware of yourself. This is a book I would recommend to clients."
~Jane Schmidt, founder of Parent Coaching NW, LLC, Seattle, WA.

"I am struck by how wise and wonderful this book is. So much self-care is nurtured and suggested, here...I wish I'd had it when I was young, but I'm glad to read it now, glad younger women get to know and have this wonderful resource."
~Naomi Rose, editor, book developer,
creator of *Writing From the Deeper Self*, Oakland, CA.

"This book plants seeds. Each woman can find what appeals to her. It is very refreshing, with humor, lots of information, and many helpful suggestions for how to use it. You have so much experience to share."
~Kate Markham, educational administrator, Bellingham, WA.

"Barbara, your work is a blessing to girls and women alike."
~Rachael Jean Harper, CH, NTP
Holistic Nutritional Therapist, manufacturer of the finest handcrafted, award-winning superfood

"This is a whole new paradigm!"
~Linda Bark PhD, RN
Master Certified Coach (ICF), Bark Coaching Institute, San Francisco Bay Area

"This is a very accessible, simple yet powerful set of tools…especially for women who have had difficult periods for years and need a fresh, healing and holistic perspective on this topic."
~Emily Burger, Luna Touch Bodywork, Ojai, CA.

"When I read that there have been times of honoring women's cycles and magical gifts, then I want that to happen for me! And sharing this with our daughters, so they can know some of the sacredness of their cycles, is priceless."
~Sharon, CPA, Portland, OR.

"This book has heart."
~Doug, longtime friend, Santa Barbara, CA.

Please Note: The information contained in this book is provided for educational purposes only and is not intended to be a substitute for professional medical advice. Always check with your health care provider about any questions you may have regarding a medical condition.

Welcome

You are probably reading this book because you or someone you care about would like to have an easier time with your menstrual cycle. You may be struggling with physical or emotional stresses that cause you to dread "that time of the month."

Most of the usual remedies are directed at suppressing symptoms so you can just "get on with life." I'd like to show you another way to look at your entire month. Because there is another way.

Take a step back with me and take a look at the bigger picture – the world that you inhabit, with its rhythms and seasons, and also the habits and beliefs which make up your "inner world," since these affect you at least as much as your outer world does.

Once you have a better understanding of your entire cycle (the one that goes on all month long), you will find that the "difficult days" are easier to understand. You will see that, just like the seasons of the year, your month can be viewed in terms of "seasons." You can also compare your cycle to the phases of the moon.

Just as the seasons and the moon are always changing, you too probably feel very different during one week of your month than during another. This is because your cycle is always affecting you, all month long.

This may seem obvious. Yet somehow, we have been taught to act as if our cycles are not even supposed to be happening! It has come to the point where our cycles are merely tolerated, ignored as much as possible, suppressed, resented and medicated.

Does this sound like a healthy, respectful way to treat someone? Not if we want to get along with them. And yet this is how we treat our own bodies. Is it any wonder that we have trouble with our cycles? We haven't been taught how to be comfortable with them, to work with them, or to "go with the flow," so to speak.

Despite what modern culture often tells us, PMS is not an inevitable occurrence, or a "curse." Rather, it is a *symptom* of this discomfort. Symptoms are not our enemies; they have a purpose. That purpose is to get our attention when something is out of balance, so we can make adjustments before the situation gets worse. In this book, you will learn to see how your own discomfort can guide you to notice imbalances in your life, or in your world. From there, you will learn to interact with your body in a much more positive and nurturing way.

There are many wise approaches to women's health that will enable you to feel good throughout your monthly cycle. In this book you will learn about nourishing foods and herbs, calming body treatments, and empowering beliefs and traditions. You will be amazed at the variety of support that is available.

Once you have absorbed these new insights, acting on them consciously can shift your experience in a profoundly positive way. Your pre-menstrual time will become a natural part of your monthly cycle – like a season, with its own colors and rewards. You can actually get to the point where you look forward to "that time of the month!"

What You'll Find in This Guide

To help you better understand your cycle, this guide has five parts, or steps.

Part One gives an overview of the Cycles of Nature and how they can be a model for you, to help you balance your life for better health and comfort. You will see how consciously looking at the month in four parts, similar to seasons, will help you understand your own rhythms.

Part Two offers support for "Inner Self Care:" looking after your own feelings and needs during your pre-menstrual and menstrual times – the natural times or "seasons" of the month for catching up with yourself. You will learn how to develop personal rituals and practices for living comfortably with your cycle, and ways to honor the energy levels and interests you have at different times during your cycle.

Part Three shows you a variety of ways to pamper yourself with "Outer Self–Care:" body treatments, herbs and nutrition, and paying attention to creating a healthy environment.

In **Part Four**, we step back to look at the "Bigger Picture," considering cultural attitudes. There are many cultures that honor women's cycles. As we also look at the effects of cultures that do not, you will have an opportunity to consider how this has affected YOU. It brings you full–circle back to yourself, and gives you the chance to take another look at your own beliefs about menstruation.

Finally, **Part Five** helps you to re-consider and re-imagine your own coming of age as a girl. Taking a compassionate review of your own life can help you break free of limitations you didn't even know you had, for a dramatic improvement in health, self–esteem and empowerment.

At the end of each chapter there is a Summary to help you remember the key points, followed by an Activity so that you really begin to absorb these concepts. To help you in this process there is also a sheet at the end of each chapter called "I Want to Remember," which you can use as you read to jot down anything that especially interests you. When you get to the Activity section, you can refer to that sheet so your experience of the activities is totally relevant to your interests and concerns.

This guide will show you many nurturing ways to support better health in various aspects of your life. There are many ways to find balance, and here you will have the opportunity to see what appeals to you. The main goal is to become *conscious* of your cycle, so you know what is true for you from one week to the next and how to interpret this in a positive way!

I wish you the very best. You deserve to feel proud of your miraculous, life-giving body.

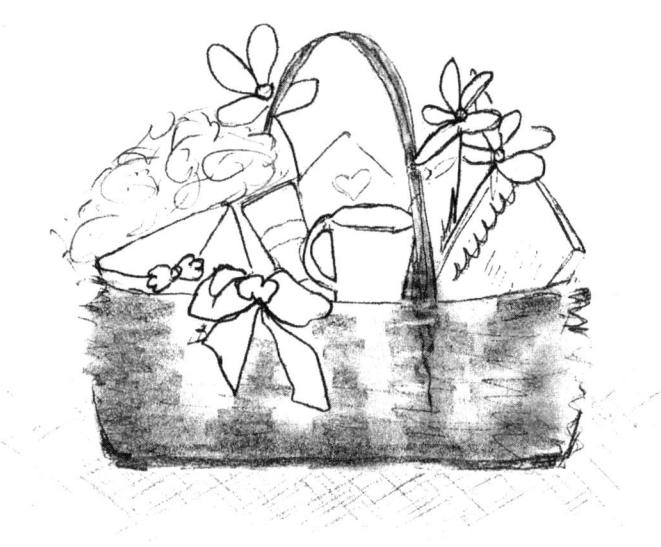

Table of Contents

Part 1: The Cycles of Nature and You..................................9
    Moon Cycle Diagram: Compare Your Own Cycle to the Moon Cycle
    Seasonal Cycle Diagram: Compare Your Own Cycle to the Seasons
    PMS is at the End of Your Cycle: What This Means
        The Imbalance Indicated by Pre-Menstrual Symptoms
    Summary
    Activity

Part 2: Caring for Your Inner Life: Developing Your Rhythm..................31
    Creative Activities to Support Your Month:
        Have Special Things to do During Your Period
        Keep a Simple Journal and Calendar
        Observe the Moon
        Take Time for Yourself
        Anticipate your Needs as Pre-menstrual Time Approaches:
        Negotiating for Time Alone
        Tears
        Sensitivity
        Speaking Your Truth
    Summary
    Activity
    Calendar Activity Pages

Part 3: Caring for Your Outer Life: Nourishing Your Body..................71
    What Kinds of Foods are Nourishing?
    Things to Consider When Deciding What to Eat
    Specific Foods
    Things to Consider Avoiding

Herbs to Consider
   Supplements
   Aromatherapy
   Healthy Habits: Light, Motion, and Rest
   Healthy Self–Care: Body Treatments
   Help for Cramps
   Alternative Menstrual Products
   Summary
   Activity

Part 4: The Big Picture: The Beliefs that Shape Cultures........................107
   Cultural Respect for Women's Cycles
   Your Own "Moon Lodge"
   Modern Culture's Disregard for Women's Cycles
   Summary
   Activity
   Red Tent Activity Pages

Part 5: Welcoming Yourself into Womanhood...............................129
   What Was Your First Period Like?
   Give Yourself the Welcome You Deserve
      Tell Your Story the Way it Was
      Tell Your Story the Way You Wish it had Been
      Give Yourself Recognition for Becoming a Woman
   Share a New Tradition With Your Daughter
   Summary
   Activity

Author's Note

References and Additional Resources...151
    Part 1: The Cycles of Nature and You
    Part 2: Caring for Your Inner Life
    Part 3: Caring for Your Outer Life
    Part 4: The Big Picture
    Part 5: Welcoming Yourself into Womanhood
    Complete Book List
    Additional Recommended Reading
    Recommended Resources

Tamara Slayton – an Inspiration

About the Author

Acknowledgements

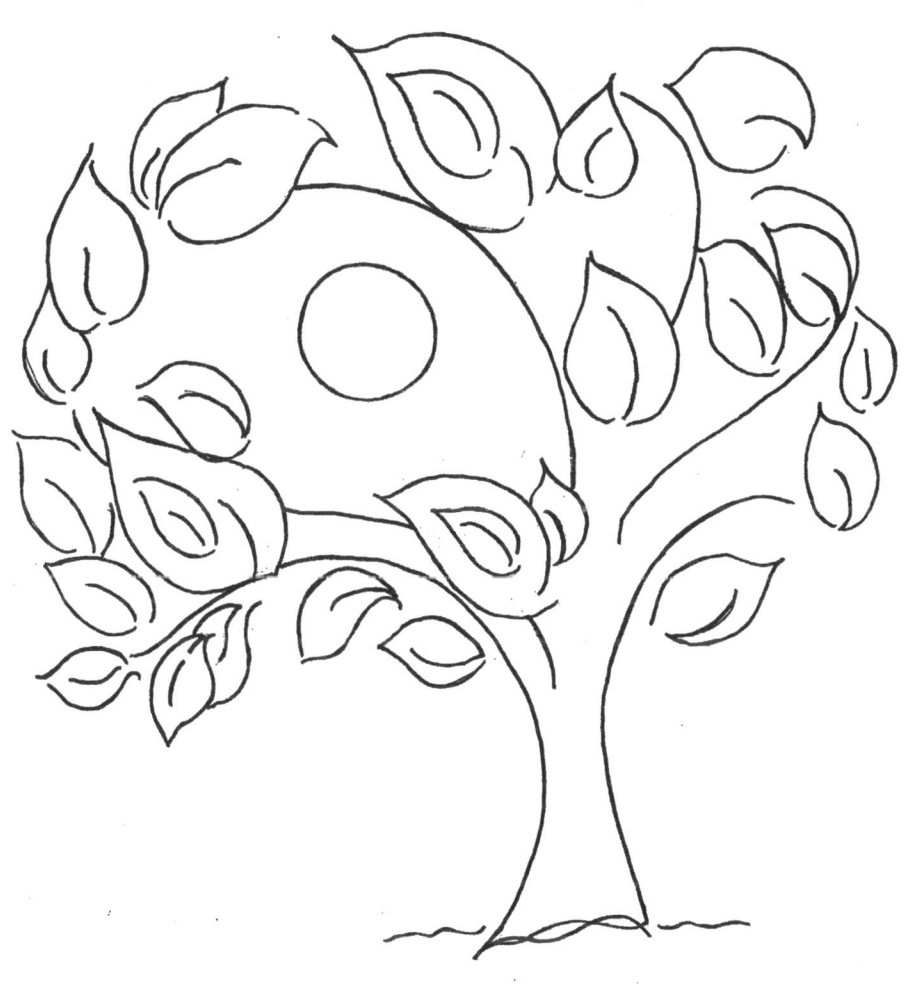

Part 1

The Cycles of Nature and You

"We can turn to our bodies to experience our connection to Nature."
~Judith Lasater

When I was five, I made up a little song about the seasons, and sang it to my grandmother. Recently I found that song, faintly written in pencil in my grandmother's hand, on a faded sheet of paper. It touched my heart that she had recorded that moment, and to think of myself as a five-year-old, already enchanted by the seasons: little did I know how that theme would carry through my life!

For as long as I can remember, I've pictured the year as a circle, with summer at the top and winter at the bottom. The symbol of the circle is common to all cultures as the Circle of Life, coming "full circle" and beginning again, over and over.

This simple, universal symbol is a key for women as a monthly model for balance and self-renewal.

When you learn to visualize your month as a circle, not only will you know where you are and where you're going that month, you will also see how you fit into other, larger cycles of life as well. You will begin to feel that you belong. You fit. You fit with the themes that are eternal.

And that has always been true. Older, more Indigenous cultures, have always seen the menstrual cycle in this way. It is only modern culture that has lost its way. In Part 4 we will look at how natural cycles have been valued in different cultures. Respect for the cycles of nature tends to translate into respect for the cycles of women; some cultures honor cycles far more than others.

In modern culture, however, we may just tolerate our periods, dread our pre-menstrual days, and ignore the rest! When we become conscious of the concept of the whole circle, it is like pulling back a veil and becoming aware of what else is going on when we're not paying any attention. Then, the whole picture is revealed – and it all makes sense.

"Waking up" to our cycle means learning to notice where we are in our cycle, so we can plan ahead and anticipate our needs, preparing for our continual changes as we would prepare for the seasons. Then we're in harmony with our own rhythms. Since they affect everything in our lives...everything starts to go better.

Let's begin by talking about the month.

What does it mean to have a cycle that has different phases all month long? The phases are always flowing from one to the next: from darkness comes the light of a new beginning, which turns into bright expression, wanes into completion, and then back to the slumber of darkness—the seeds of new beginning.

> "In contemporary society, with the realities of working, traveling, and all the possibilities for distraction and entertainment that are regularly set before our eyes, it's difficult to realize that a vast, orderly universe exists all around us, operating according to an infinitely structured, almost symphonic rhythm. We may try to ignore that rhythm, but it still asserts itself even through the static of everyday life."
> ~Deepak Chopra, *Restful Sleep*.

What can you expect from your cycle as it fluctuates through the month, and how can you learn more about your own rhythms? How can you learn to think of them in a positive way?

NATURE'S MODEL OF BALANCE

The cycles of nature provide us with a model – a model of balance: light balances dark, activity is balanced by rest. This model will be your guide for appreciating and anticipating your own needs, as you approach your cycle with a new understanding, and greatly ease your discomfort.

Even though "balance" is a term that is over-used these days, nature shows us the real thing. By looking at nature we can see that true balance does not mean trying to juggle everything at once. Rather, it is about seasons. We might as well accept the season we're in, knowing that the others will come around again in their own time.

When you notice stress in your health or your emotions (which is more likely to come up pre-menstrually), you will know to look for ways to bring yourself back into harmony, remembering which season you're in, and thus taking good care of yourself.

Your cycle, therefore, is your friend! It shows you when things are getting off-kilter in your life.

THE PHASES OF THE MOON

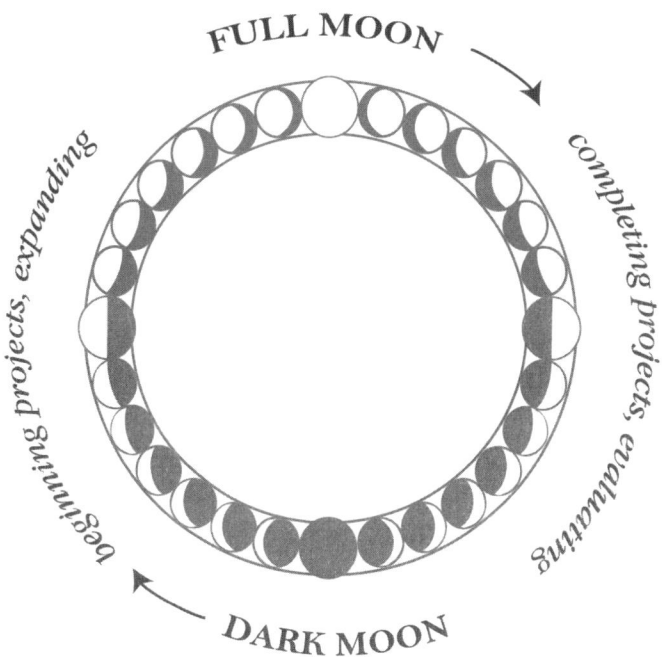

"The ancients called the dark days of the moon 'woman's moon' or 'resting moon,' linking a woman's physical, emotional and spiritual state to the lunar wheel."
~Maya Tiwari

The illustration above shows the moon's cycle, as it goes from dark to full. The diagram also represents the phases of a woman's monthly cycle, and suggests how best to use these energies in your life. Growing light supports expanding energy, while waning light suggests completion.

The Full Moon, which is easily visible each month, is a bright, expressive time. You are undoubtedly familiar with the Full Moon; but you may not be familiar with Dark Moon. This is an equally powerful phase of the moon, corresponding to a powerful part of a woman's cycle.

Dark Moon occurs on the night before New Moon, the night when there is no moon at all – the opposite of Full Moon. Dark Moon is a powerful time of inward focus, inner power, and potential, in contrast with the radiance and expansion of Full Moon.

I think of Dark Moon as a "Still Point" – a pause before the cycle begins again. Like the pause after you exhale and before you take the next breath, when everything feels just still. It is a potent state of "being," rather than "doing."

Compare Your Own Cycle to the Moon Cycle

It's so helpful to realize that the moon actually provides guidance for optimizing women's own "phases of the moon." Once you learn to recognize it, you will have a built-in regulator for your own well-being right at hand.

Women's cycles, as you probably know, are similar to the moon's. In fact, this connection is so strong that women who live much of their life in nature, out under the sky, find that their menstrual cycles often come into synchronicity with the moon's cycles fairly quickly. Irregular menstruation can even be made more regular by paying attention to the moon. (You'll find more suggestions for this in Part 2.)

Women's bodies respond to the moon on two levels: we have a physical cycle, and we also have an inner energetic cycle which reflects the moon's path through the month.

This inner cycle is what has been forgotten in modern culture. The good news is that when we remember this inner rhythm, we remember how to guide ourselves through the month without burning out!

You have your own "Full Moon" each month, at ovulation, and your own "Dark Moon" each month, at menstruation.

Typically, a woman's energy will be more like the growing and full moon after her period, until after ovulation: expanding outward, beginning projects, enthusiastic, focused on others, more social, and more optimistic. Then, after the cycle has peaked, it turns downward again.

Pre-menstrual and menstrual energies are more like the waning and dark moon. The energy is drawing inward, back toward the center. This is the time when you are naturally drawn back to yourself, to focus on your own feelings and needs.

This time of drawing inward is a natural balance to all the energy that a woman usually spends focusing on other people. The only problem is that modern culture does not support this need of women to turn inward for renewal once a month.

However, *you* can choose to make room for this inner renewal. And once you start working with these concepts, you will see that there is a natural balance to your month, and another, more supportive way to interpret your pre-menstrual upsets. In other words, if you are irritable pre-menstrually, it may not be that your hormones are "out of balance," but rather that they are doing their job of signaling you (loudly?!) that it is time to take care of yourself and take your own needs seriously. **When you don't pay attention to this signal, it gets louder.**

The problem is not with you. It is with the culture that has lost the meaning and value of cycles, leaving you struggling to understand and accept your own experience – and often lacking support to do so.

You can learn to support your own need for this different, internal focus. The regularity of the moon's passage through the month can be a reminder to you that these are totally natural changes for you as well – part of the flow of energy from within to without, and back again. Each sustains the other.

As you learn to respect your body, it will nourish and support you. Your body and brain will be thankful for:

- rest when they crave rest;
- healthy food when they crave certain nutrients;
- play when they need spontaneous, non-structured activity.
- A run around the block? A walk with the neighbor's dog? Some puttering in the yard? Fifteen minutes with a coloring book or a ball? Something you've been wanting to do but don't think you have the time?

How about doing just a little bit, for a few minutes? You will feel more cared for and stronger, and some of the internal discomforts designed to get your attention may ease. Aches and pains may diminish. Sleep may improve. New ideas and solutions may arise spontaneously. Laughter may find its way to the surface more often.

> "If you are willing to court the rhythmical life of your body you are given access to something Other that happens naturally. And the very act of courting the inner life of your body itself builds an inner sweetness, surety and dignity – a spirit of sovereign authority that is priceless."
> ~Alexandra Pope, *The Woman's Quest.*

The main thing is that as you pay more attention you will be learning about your cycle and treating it as if it were important – because it is! You will find your own ways of working with the different phases of your month. And if your way of finding balance and navigating your month turns out to be totally different than someone else's, that's just fine. You are a unique human being, after all.

> "The menstrual cycle governs the flow not only of fluids but of information and creativity. Astrologer Sioux Rose refers to this as our moon dance - our initiation into the feminine dimensions of time. We receive and process information differently at different times in our cycles."
>
> "Since our culture generally appreciates only what we can understand rationally, many women tend to block at every opportunity the flow of unconscious "lunar" information that comes to them pre-menstrually or during their menstrual cycle. Lunar information…comes to us in our dreams, our emotions, our hungers. It comes under cover of darkness…the luteal phase, from ovulation until the onset on menstruation, is when women are most in tune with their inner knowing and with what isn't working in their lives."
>
> "Society is not nearly as keen on this as it is on the follicular phase. Thus we judge our pre-menstrual energy, emotions and inward mood as 'bad' and 'unproductive.'"
> ~Dr. Christiane Northrup, *Women's Bodies, Women's Wisdom.*

THE SEASONS

You can see how other cycles of nature can fit the same circular model. Below is the same moon diagram, this time with the seasons of the year added around the circle.

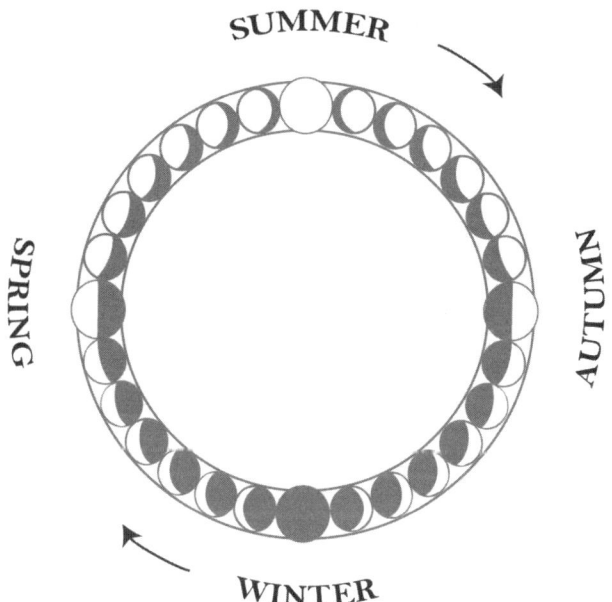

Compare Your Own Cycle to the Seasons

When you look at the seasons of the year, you can clearly see the same flow of energy as with the moon, as the seasons move from one to the next. Spring begins the new year of growth, followed by the brightness of Summer, and the harvest of Autumn. Winter completes the year, when many plants go inward and draw back down into their roots.

Season 1: Green Shoots, new energy. Springtime. **Beginning, expanding**.

Season 2: Full Bloom, radiant energy. Summer. **Above ground, outward.**

Season 3: Harvest, returning energy. Autumn. **Completion, evaluation.**

Season 4: Roots, resting energy. Winter. **Below ground, open inwardly.**

In comparing the seasons to the moon cycle, you can see that Summer is like the full moon – bright and full of energy. Winter is more like the dark moon – a time of rest, with longer nights. Your own ovulation time corresponds with the full moon and summer, when you are likely to be more focused on others. The approach of your menstrual time corresponds with the waning and dark moon, or winter, when the light dims and draws inward.

Cycles are all around you and within you. They are how nature works – and you are no exception. Even a breath, just a single breath, is a simple yet powerful example of filling up and expanding, and then releasing and coming back to the starting point.

> "I enjoy thinking of my body as not only parallel to, but part of, the seasons. It makes everything we go through feel purposeful, even the discomfort."
> ~Emily Burger, Luna Touch Bodywork, Ojai, CA.

The simple truth of the need for balance is native to *us,* but not to our culture. We simply have not been taught to honor this need in ourselves. And it is the resulting neglect of our basic nature – not anything "wrong" with us – that causes such stress in our health, our self-esteem, and our quality of life.

Think of trees. In spring, trees are fresh with new leaves. In summer, they are full and expressive with leaves and fruit. In autumn, the leaves fall all around in blazing, colorful harvest. And in winter, most trees lose their leaves, pull inward, drawing their energy down into their roots, and go underground. Does this mean that they are sick, or lazy, or unreliable? Of course not. They are drawing energy into their roots so they will have something to *give*, as they emerge into their coming year with full focus and enthusiasm.

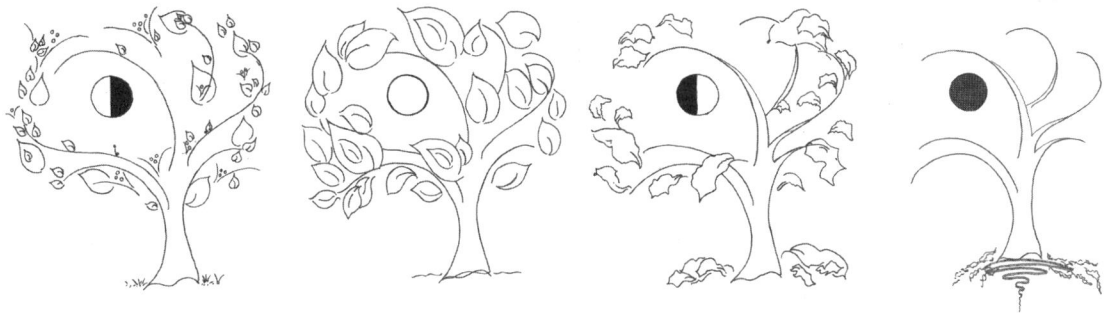

PMS IS AT THE END OF YOUR CYCLE; WHAT THIS MEANS

"Often, pre-menstrual tension is an expression of built-up resentment over not doing what really inspires you."
~Karin C. Uphoff

Pre-menstrual syndrome happens in the equivalent of Season 3, Autumn, as you approach the end of your monthly cycle. This same time of the month that causes so much distress is actually designed as a healing time!

Season 3 is the Harvest; time to **reflect and learn the meaning** of what has gone on the rest of the month. During the "outward" weeks, before and during ovulation, it is easier to stay busy and focused on tasks and other people. Living more on the surface, it is easier to get a lot done, but it is also easier to breeze right by the impact or meaning of events.

The focus now, in season 3, is all about returning to self, evaluating, fixing what is out of balance, reflecting on your month, and receiving what you need...just like the trees.

This is time to care for yourself. The end of the cycle means it is important to put things in order. This is Autumn, the time of drawing inward, making everything ready for winter, *evaluating* to see what serves you and what is no longer needed.

The pre-menstrual time is a powerful personal time: visionary, creative, and inwardly focused. This is in direct conflict, of course, with the expectations of modern culture for constant accomplishment, and for women to be always available and accommodating of others.

You can see why this causes us some difficulties! And yet once we begin to interpret things differently, a lot of the difficulties will take care of themselves. For example, if you are irritable, does that mean your hormones are out of balance? Or could it mean that you have been insanely busy for three weeks and need a break? If you cry more easily, does it mean you are "too sensitive?" Or that you are expressing the tension that your body needs to release? If you don't want to spend time with a friend, does it mean that you are selfish? Or are you just realizing that you need a night off to recharge?

The menstrual time that follows pre-menstruation also becomes a stressful and uncomfortable condition when the culture requires women to be pleasing, compliant and available all

> "Simply being in touch with the cycle has its own quiet magic and inner sweetener for our lives. At first it may be barely noticeable, but if you can sustain the process of attention you'll be building an inner sanctum...by this I mean a respect for yourself that casts its glow everywhere. This is the basic spiritual practice for your menstruating years."
> ~Alexandra Pope, *The Woman's Quest.*

the time. This just isn't the way cycles work – not the moon's, not the seasons', and not women's.

Since the menstrual time reflects winter, this is a time for becoming more still (in a way that feels right for you), in order to listen to the larger messages of your life that can get lost in all the noise of daily activity.

Or...just to take a bubble bath with no one knocking at the door!

The Imbalance Indicated by Pre-Menstrual Symptoms

If you have pre-menstrual discomfort or symptoms, this is not something to accept as inevitable. This is a signal to you that something is "off." PMS is a signal of imbalance, and it is there for a reason – to get you to pay attention and take care of whatever has come to the surface.

What kind of imbalance is it?

Conventionally, the types of imbalances addressed have to do with nutrition or hormones. Yet, while it is true that it could be a hormonal imbalance (some women feel better when they take hormonal supplements) or a nutritional need (for more or less of something), this is only part of the story. For you are *at least* as affected by stresses to your emotions and your spirit as you are by imbalances on the physical level.

When you are pre-menstrual you see things in a different way. We have been trained to think there is something wrong with us at this time, but it may be that we simply don't understand the real message of our discomfort. Therefore, instead of dismissing our discomfort, we need to look for the truth within it.

For example:

- we may feel desperate for some time to ourselves, or;
- to be more creative, or;
- to be taken more seriously.
- Your body could be reacting to past traumas that it still holds.
- You could be deeply troubled by conditions in the larger world, as well.
- And, as if that weren't enough, your experience of your cycle is imprinted by what you have been told about menstruation, ever since you were a girl.

> "My experience of my own menstrual cycle began to change after I noticed that my most meaningful insights about myself, my life, and my writing came on the day or two just before my period. In my mid-thirties, I began to look forward to my periods, understanding them to be sacred time that our culture didn't honor."
> ~Dr. Christiane Northrup, *Women's Bodies, Women's Wisdom.*

This kind of "inner knowing" is more accessible when we are pre-menstrual, which is when these feelings surface. And so the reason it is so important to treat the "whole person" (and not just a symptom) is that if your distress stems from deeper causes such as these, treating the physical body will only bring temporary relief. Listening to your own body and mind, rather than what you have picked up from the culture, is what will lead you to healing. Your wise and intuitive body and mind know, and want to let *you* know, when something is not right.

This time of release and reckoning, at the end of your cycle, is a time for righting what is wrong, so that the new cycle can begin from the best perspective. This end-of-cycle time is where wisdom and experience are nourished. This is where you pause to reflect in order to find the meaning of your experiences, see what needs to be changed, and plan how to fix things.

You don't even have to know how to do this, at this point. It's enough to realize that your internal cycle provides for your maximum well-being, once you start working with it. In the following chapters, we will go more deeply into all these aspects of your well-being.

Your discomforts can be addressed, soothed and improved, at a pace that feels right for you.

So, let's begin to look at ways you can bring more balance to your life!

> Remembering the balance of nature is a way to realize that there is a rhythm to life. There are seasons, with each season having its own priorities. You cannot rush seasons. Better to fully open to them, dwell within them and find their natural pace...to see what needs to be grown, enjoyed, gathered, studied, or left alone for another time. By stepping into your cycle, you will come home to the natural balance that will keep you healthy and fulfilled.

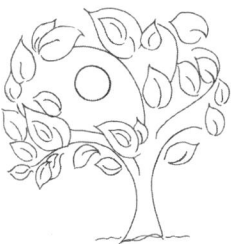

SUMMARY

Throughout the natural world, on earth and out into the cosmos, cycles are the way things work. Cycles have a movement, then a rest. Waves of energy work in a similar way – waves of water, light or sound all travel by pulses of energy, generating new energy by pausing before continuing. This pause gives the push, or momentum, to the next wave.

It is self-defeating, even harmful, for women to try to suppress this powerful and sustaining source of energy within. Your monthly cycle is a complete inner journey each month through the four seasons. By observing and allowing this flow – by coming back to your center, each month – you have a place from which to launch the next cycle for your best outcome. When you do this, you will be replenished instead of exhausted – inspired instead of resentful!

The time of pre-menstruation is Season 3; the time of harvest, completion and evaluation. It is a time to pay attention to your own feelings and needs. Your energy is naturally drawing inward, to encourage you to reflect on where you have been and to nourish you for where you are going.

This is the time when you are alerted to what needs your attention. Your body has a wise design, and discomfort has meaning.

Deeper issues, thoughts and feelings come to the surface when you are pre-menstrual. Things that have gone unresolved want your attention.

These could be:

- Things about your body and outer life, such as nutrition, exercise, and environment.
- Things about your relationships and your inner world, such as need for time alone, self-expression, fulfillment and creativity.
- You could be reacting to long-ago traumas that still live in your body.
- You could be reacting to troubling issues in the larger world which call to your caring nature and sense of justice.

Your pre-menstrual time is a time for telling the truth (or – to put it another way – a time when the truth tells itself!) In the following chapters, you will learn how to give the truth – *your* truth – space to be heard; to relate to it in a new way and to act on it for the best outcome.

ACTIVITY:

You will find very simple activities after each chapter. Doing these will ensure that you really begin to absorb these concepts.

To step into the model of the moon and seasons, visualize your month as a circle, with ovulation at the top, and menstruation at the bottom. Drawing it will help you to visualize it more easily:

- Draw a circle on a piece of paper;
- Draw a full moon at the top of the circle and a dark moon at the bottom;
- Now add the words "ovulation" to the top, and "menstruation" to the bottom.

This seems simple, but doing it will help you integrate these concepts. Add words, decorations, or colors if you want!

(There are sample pages of charts and calendars later in this book, at the end of Part 2, for you to use each month as you develop these concepts further.)

I WANT TO REMEMBER:

As you read this chapter, jot down anything here that especially interests you; things you especially want to remember, or ideas that occur to you as you read. This page will help you reflect on these things you notice at more length, and think them through a little more or come back to them later.

I Want to Remember:

_____

_____

_____

_____

_____

_____

_____

_____

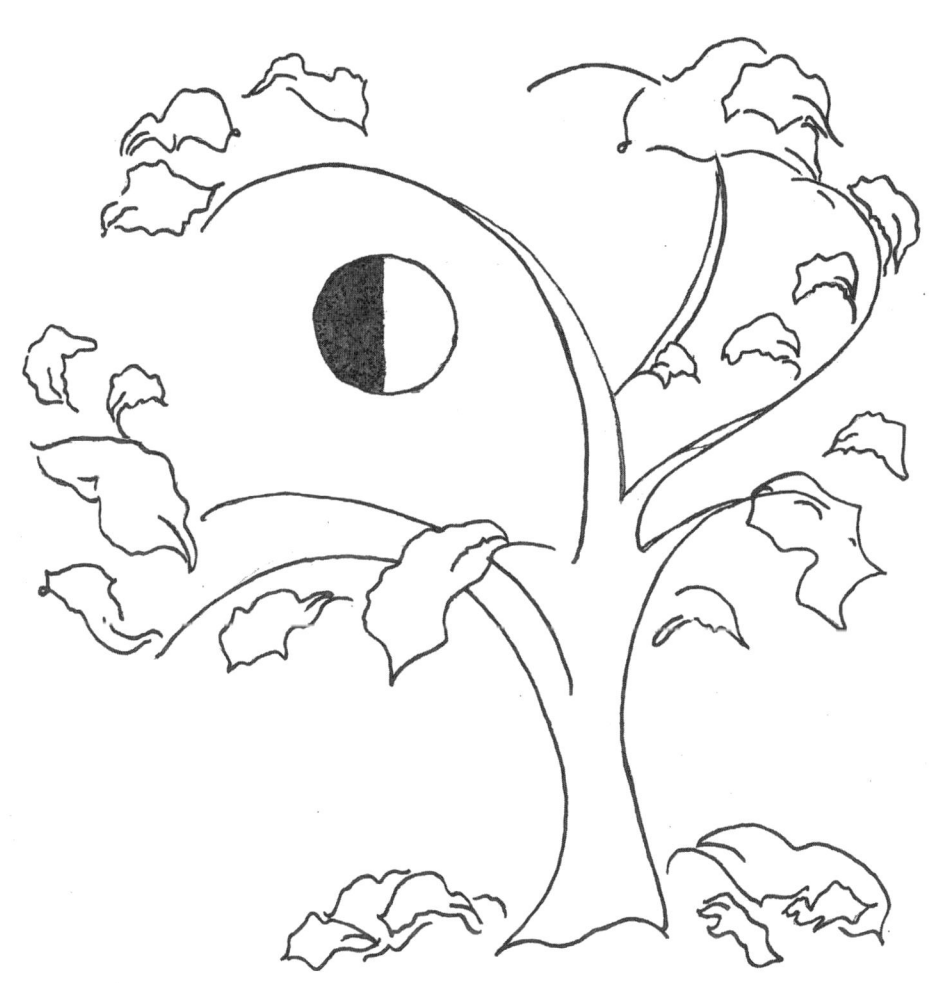

Part 2

Caring for Your Inner Life: Developing Your Rhythm

"How right it is to work my wonders in the world, empowered by the chant within."
~Danaan Parry

Let us now go more deeply into how to integrate your cycle into your life, so you can support yourself and feel better all month long.

CREATIVE ACTIVITIES TO SUPPORT YOUR MONTH

Here are five ways to help you understand and support your cycle. We'll go through these one at a time.

- Have special things to do during your period.
- Keep a simple journal and calendar.
- Observe the moon's cycle.
- Take time for yourself.
- Anticipate your needs as pre-menstrual time approaches.

Have Special Things to Do During Your Period

A good way to begin to honor your cycle is to do something special when your period starts each month. Begin to imagine what these could be...pleasant things that you will look forward to.

The main point is, this is a time when your energy turns inward toward yourself, toward your own feelings and needs. It's a time for renewing and supporting yourself; replenishing your energy.

What does this mean to you? How can you support yourself? You can do simple things, just to let yourself know that you are noticing what's going on as you go about your day; it can be like a little wink or secret signal to yourself. A special bracelet, a favorite scarf that you only bring out at this time, some secret red power underwear!

(In fact, Lisa Sarasohn, author of the *Woman's Belly Book*, suggests that you decorate some of your underwear with power symbols. "Consider the ways in which your belly serves you...and create a pair of undies that honors your belly in style!")

You could also have a pretty box to bring out. This is a beautiful tradition, in which women create a hatbox or basket for themselves that they bring out each month for their personal time, full of nurturing things that they find special.

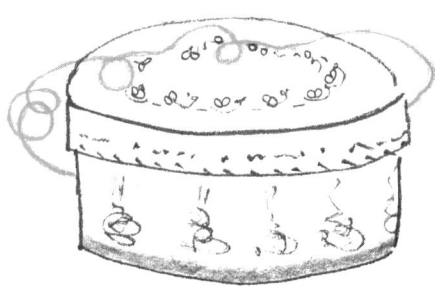

A journal and pen, items with appealing textures and colors, luscious towels, scarves, candles, teas. A special mug. A bracelet, a poem, a stone. Create your box and have it be a gift for yourself each month. Really make it as beautiful as you can, and you will feel honored.

> When I first met Tamara Slayton, my mentor in this work, in Sebastopol, CA, she was teaching these concepts to women from around the country, and giving lovely celebrations to welcome girls who were entering puberty. Tamara introduced beauty to the concept of women's cycles, and wove them together in a timeless tapestry with the rhythms of nature and larger celestial patterns, similar to the framework in this book.
>
> We deserve to have meaning and beauty associated with our experience as females! Without the cycle of life within us, humans would not exist! It is time for us to re-imagine this whole process, and make it one that serves us. ~BH

Here are some other ideas:

- Get your bare feet onto the earth. Spend time in nature. Lean with your back against a tree and just breathe deeply for awhile. This is very calming.
- Allow room for creativity. There may be a powerful urge to express yourself. Have some of your favorite materials handy. *The Creative Journal* and other books by Lucia Capaccione have many simple ideas for drawing and collage – no experience necessary!
- Once your period begins, look at your calendar for the next month and put a red line through several of the days, at the approximate time that you think your main days of inner focus will be happening again. This way, you can plan to keep those days free of outer–focused activities as much as possible. Then, when the time comes, you can decide what you want to do – and what you don't. Don't schedule the dentist! Don't cram your days full to the brim! Leave time free just for yourself.

- Work out a trade with other women, so that you can give each other a few hours off by taking over each others' duties when it would be most appreciated. Older women who are no longer menstruating, or women on a different cycle than yours, would be ideal.

These activities are personal rituals, in that they are "markers." By taking note of certain days or moments in your life, you give yourself the message that you notice what is happening and consider it important.

Keep a Simple Journal and Calendar

One of the best ways to start having a conscious cycle and helping your month to go more smoothly is to keep some kind of calendar, chart and journal all month long, in order to learn more about your own patterns of behavior during the month. These records can be very simple.

First, keep a calendar to simply mark the days of your period each month. This will help you anticipate the arrival of your next period, as well as begin to keep a record of your own rhythm. (You'll find special calendar pages at the end of this chapter which can be printed out at http://www.womenswaymooncycles.com/calendar.html)

> "I used to wonder, 'why am I so tired? What's wrong with me?' Now I can look at my calendar and give myself permission to go take a nap."
> ~Kim, Health Care Practitioner.

Then, begin to keep a more detailed chart. This still won't take much time. (A sample annual chart is located at the end of the chapter, as well.) You can notate all sorts of things here, even making up your own "code" of symbols for different things you want to record. And once you start to pay attention, you will notice more.

Finally, have a journal alongside this chart, where you can record some of your observations more fully.

To keep the chart, you will record "Day 1" on the first day of menstruation. On this chart, you can then keep track of the differences you notice in yourself from one week to the next in terms of things like:

- Energy level,
- How your body feels,
- How social you feel,
- How happy or sad you feel, etc.

You can take note of:

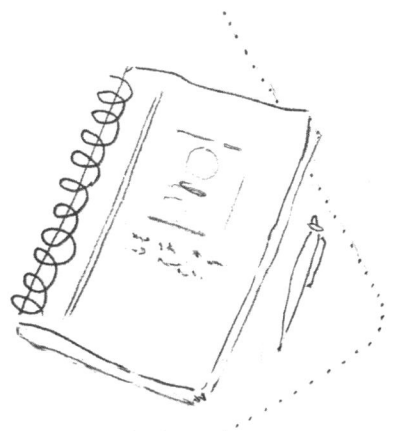

- How deeply you feel certain emotions,
- How much sleep your body wants and the quality of sleep you get,
- What colors appeal to you,
- What foods you crave,
- How you dress,
- How you relate to others.

You might find patterns in:

- How easily you argue,
- Whether you feel easily upset,
- Whether you spend time in nature,
- What you dream about…

The possibilities are endless.

Notice the inspirations you get, the ideas that come to you. Record them. You may find special intuition and ideas popping in during your period, since it is a visionary time.

During the days of your period, notice what your menstrual flow is like. Then you can notice any differences from month to month, and also learn what your typical pattern is. Notice the flow each day:

- Which days are heavier,
- What time of day is heaviest,
- How long your period lasts,
- How your body feels.

When you write things down you will be more likely to notice the connection between what is going on in your life and how your period may respond to that.

Notice when you ovulate, too, and what it feels like. Record your "fertile flow" – the clear flow that comes when you are ovulating. When you menstruate, your flow is red, of course. After menstruation, there will be no flow for awhile. And then you will notice fertile flow.

> Become interested in the quality and quantity of both your menstrual flow and fertile flow: "Ovulation flow is as important as the blood, as an indication of how prana [energy] is or isn't moving in the reproductive organs".
> ~Kellen Brugman, Yoga Teacher and Ayurvedic Lifestyle Counselor, Santa Barbara, CA.

Following Tamara Slayton's example, I say "flow" instead of "discharge," because "discharge" implies that something is wrong. Nothing is wrong! You are a beautiful, fertile, fluid female. Every female can learn to identify the signs of her own fertility and become self-aware and educated. This is helpful whether you want to become pregnant, avoid pregnancy, or just be assured that your body is operating normally. For more on ovulation and fertile flow, please see page 68.

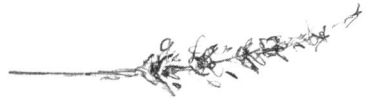

This is how you become wise: by paying attention to your own experience as if it is important, and observing it to find its meaning for you! Be present to your own life!

Stop all the distractions for awhile and notice how you are doing. That is what your cycle is inviting you to do.

Your hormones invite you into different states of consciousness throughout the month. Each of these states has its own value. Ovulation is usually a more social and pleasing time, while menstruation brings deeper awareness, such as deep insights and "aha" moments. Notice when these happen for you and record them. You may begin to see a pattern.

> For a more in-depth and creative look at the monthly dance of female hormones, take a look at the wonderful work of Marina Alzugaray's "My Moon Cards," or the book, *Cycles of Life: A Journal for Women*, by Ashley Ross.
>
> Here is an evocative example from Marina's "My Moon Cards:"
>
> "Red is for your period. Blue represents water, the wet growing time of your cycle before ovulation. Gold represents ovulation, when you lay your golden egg…"
>
> You can see that Marina is very creative and colorful in her work!

Loving Your Lady Parts

[Edited for length from the TEDx talk by Alisa Vitti, functional nutritionist and founder of FLO Living Center, http://www.floliving.com. Alisa has helped thousands of women with the five-step nutritional protocol she developed to support the endocrine system and has launched the first women's digital health care program; the FLO Hormonal Synchronization System.™]

"If we can become fluent in the language of our bodies, we can have access to an infinite source of energy, vitality, clarity, and unwavering purpose.

In the **Follicular Phase** [after menstruation], you have the most access to creative energy. Effortlessly. This is the perfect time to begin new projects.

In the **Ovulation Phase**, you have the best communication skills and the most energy that you will have all month. This is the perfect time to have important conversations. Wouldn't it be genius if you could plan to ask for a raise when you're ovulating? You're irresistible!

In the **Luteal Phase** [after ovulation], you become very detail oriented. That shoe closet you've been wanting to organize? It's very easy to do, now.

In the **Menstrual Phase**, you have the most conversation between the right and left hemispheres of your brain. If you want to course-correct or evaluate your life, this would be the time to do it. Pay attention to those gut-feeling body messages.

These important physical structures in our bodies [our endocrine system] give us this blueprint for how to organize our lives. Women in our culture have not been taught this. But if you adhere to the map, it's all laid out for you. You don't need to push or struggle.

Gloria Steinem once said that girls are taught to view their bodies as unending projects to work on, whereas boys from a young age are taught to view their bodies as tools to master their environment.

Unfortunately, the environment is mastering us right now. Women's bodies are in hormonal breakdown in epidemic proportions. When you learn how to eat to support your body, and plan your month thematically, week over week in accordance with these hormonal ratios, you, too, can leverage your body as a "power tool.""

www.FloLiving.com

Observe the Moon

> *"Spending time outdoors, immersed in the natural world, will help your mind settle into the miracle of your own existence."*
> ~Karin C. Uphoff

When you also observe the moon on the chart you are keeping, you will become much more conscious of how everything fits together! You will see what phase the moon is in when you are menstruating or ovulating, and you will naturally become more aware of the moon's rhythm as you follow your own rhythm. You may even see them begin to synchronize with each other. You may also notice a different quality to your menstrual days, depending on what phase the moon is in. For example, if you are menstruating at dark moon, the two cycles are both at their depth at the same time, so you may find yourself being drawn internally to an even greater degree.

One month I found myself menstruating at dark moon, and it was also during the darkest time of the year. I was aware of the three cycles lining up, like three big wheels coming together—and I was at the bottom of them all! I felt hazy and unfocused. But rather than trying to fight it, I went into it.

I reminded myself that one of the qualities of darkness is—you cannot see! So I surrendered to the value that was there for me. I gave up any attempts to figure anything out, feel better, or even to be creative. I just lay down on the floor, focused on one breath at a time, and let the floor support me. I even allowed myself to release awareness of my body, as if it could dissolve.

It was a profound lesson in trust. I recognized that I had access at that time to a wide–open space of not-knowing, and I let myself surrender to it. "Letting go" in such a way allows for deep release – so imagination, thoughts, and body patterns can loosen, and then emerge in a new way when you finally get up again!

I did create a collage, later that day, which can be seen on my web site. ~BH

Have a calendar available that shows the moon phases so that you get in the habit of knowing what phase the moon is in, as you go about your month. (See page 44 for more on where to look for the moon.) You can do this without even looking at the night sky. However—it will be very beneficial for you to notice the moon in the night sky as often as you can.

Refer to the calendar that tells you when the moon is full, and when it is dark. Make yourself as aware of the "moon's calendar" as you are of the regular calendar, as you go about your month. This is so important because the moon's cycle is a *natural* calendar. It was the first calendar, and "tuning in" to the moon helps women, especially, to come into harmony with nature around us. Keep this awareness of the moon's phases in mind until it becomes part of your inner rhythm, your inner awareness.

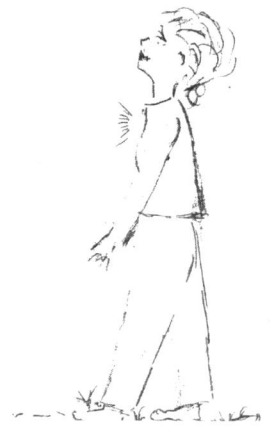

Also, as I suggested earlier, remember to actually look at the moon, occasionally. Find it in the sky, then take a minute or two to really take the moon's light into your eyes and body. It has been said that "the moon is a woman's friend." Your body will respond well to your attention to the moon. When your body knows what the moon is doing, then it can respond to the moon's rhythm. This can even regulate an irregular cycle.

If you want to align your own cycle to the moon's rhythm, so that you begin to menstruate on dark moon, try to follow these habits of knowing where the moon is in its cycle, and spending time in the moonlight. Have the conscious, loving intention of coming into alignment with the moon. Be patient with yourself, as it may take awhile to establish your new rhythm.

Another way of aligning your cycle with the moon is to create a cycle of light and dark in the room where you sleep. This method is effective for shifting your menstrual rhythm. Begin by sleeping with light in the room for a few nights during full moon, and then have total darkness for a few nights during dark moon. If you can't have the moonlight shining into your room, you could even leave a light on. Then, during dark moon, you need to be sure there are no light sources either in your room, or coming in from outside, such as streetlights. It must be totally dark, as a moonless night would be. Your body will often respond to this lunar rhythm by beginning to menstruate at the dark moon, and maintain a more regular cycle from month to month.

> "Most women report a dramatic improvement in health as soon as their menstrual cycles starts to flow in accord with the new moon."
> ~Maya Tiwari, *The Path of Practice.*

Even if your body carries on with its own unique cycle (that is, not in rhythm with the moon's), you may discover reasons for the pattern your body has or the dates it chooses. Some women find that they are bleeding on significant days that have personal meaning for them. I had two occasions when my (usually very regular) period came at very unusual times that recognized important anniversary dates in my life.

A woman may find that her period has adjusted its timing in order to adapt to challenging demands in her schedule. Try to ask for your body's cooperation in the timing of your cycle, and see what happens!

How can you tell where to look for the moon?

The full moon always rises at sunset, since it is on the opposite side of the earth from the sun. When the moon and sun are on opposite sides of the earth, we can see the sunlight that is shining onto the moon's surface. That's what makes it a "full" moon – the fact that we can see it.

moon↑   earth↑   sun↑

FULL MOON: The moon and sun are on opposite sides of the earth. So, we can see the bright side of the moon. Full moon rises in the east as the sun sets in the west, as the earth turns.

As the moon goes around the earth, we can see less and less of the part that the sun is shining upon. So when the moon gets all the way around to the other side of the earth (which it does once a month), it is near the sun (or at least it looks that way to us), and it sets at around the same time the sun sets. At this time, we cannot see the bright side at all. We only see the dark side—or, rather, we *can't* see the dark side.

For a day or two, we see no moon at all. Then the moon starts to move away from the sun again (from our perspective), and we see it as a "new" moon. The new moon will always be near the sun, and will set soon after the sun sets.

The moon makes this circle around the earth once every 29 days, which is also the common length of a woman's menstrual cycle.

If you get yourself a calendar that shows you the full moons and dark moons, and you also pay attention to the moon's position in the sky, you will become more familiar with its cycle and learn where to look for it at different times of the month. It will be like seeing a friend – "Oh, there you are! I thought I'd find you here."

Sometimes it is easy to see the moon at night. Other times, it is in the sky during the daylight hours.

Watching the full moon rise at sunset is one of my very favorite things. When I am able to put a reminder about the moonrise onto my list for the day, and get myself to a good vantage point in time to see it rise, I am in awe every single time. In fact, sometimes I have gone behind a hill after it has risen, so that it is hidden by the hill and not yet in view. Then I get to see it rise all over again!

To learn more about the moon's phases, you will find several brief articles at the Women's Way web site, www.womenswaymooncycles.com.

earth ↑   moon ↑   sun ↑

DARK MOON: The moon has moved to the other side of the earth, so we cannot see the bright side. Dark moon and the sun rise and set at the same time, as the earth turns.

For example, one woman found, that by telling her body her plans for the coming month and asking for its cooperation, her period shifted by a few days and she avoided the inconvenience of having her period while traveling. Another woman noticed that her period seemed to be timing itself so that the phases of her month corresponded to the types of challenging work that she was facing.

Take Time for Yourself

As your month draws to a close – and your inner self yearns for your attention – you may have a craving for time alone that you don't even realize is there. This is a simple yet profound need that can have great benefits, if honored in even small ways.

Time out means *uninterrupted time.* No one calling on you, checking in, or needing your attention.

Let's look at some examples.

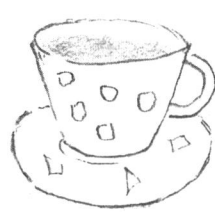

One mother found great comfort in having an evening to herself each month, curling up in her rocking chair wrapped up in a favorite quilt, listening to her favorite music, while her husband took their kids out for a few hours. Just having those hours for herself nourished her and gave her a window of time for renewal every month. And wow, did she look forward to it!

Another woman noticed she had a need for time alone every other month. It was as if one ovary needed more space than the other! She and her husband learned to honor this and anticipate her need for quiet, uninterrupted time on alternate months. Rather than getting into a fight in order to get some space, she learned to anticipate and communicate her needs. One of the things she liked to do was just retreat to her room with a good book for the evening, and no conversation.

Some women even manage to take an entire day off, with the help of friends if necessary, so they can just spend a day doing nothing in particular. (You will find more on "menstrual lodges," where women have traditionally gone during menstruation, in Part 4.)

Practically speaking, though, just small and simple changes can mean a lot. The big difference is that, in paying attention to what is happening, you are "cycling consciously" and looking for ways to support yourself. Believe me, your "inner self" will notice the attention and respond.

> This whole idea of 'time out' corresponds with the practice of honoring Sabbath each week. Many women are reclaiming the value of Sabbath as time out from normal activities. Actually, the original Sabbath occurred once a month! It was associated with women and the moon, and was a day of rest, reverie and imagination. ~BH

Here are a couple of suggestions for small and simple, yet potent, changes:

- Try talking less in order to conserve energy as you go about your day,
- Talk to a special friend, or don't talk to anyone at all.

You may be craving "time out" but not know when or how to make it happen. Now that you know you have a natural rhythm that shows you the optimal times for personal time, you can plan and anticipate your needs, and you can show others how to help you.

In the next section, we will look more carefully at how to accomplish this.

ANTICIPATING YOUR NEEDS AS PRE-MENSTRUAL TIME APPROACHES

If you don't understand and accommodate your needs at pre-menstrual time, they can be forceful and disruptive. The good news is that as you become more familiar with your cycle, you will know how to plan ahead. Here are a few things to consider:

- Negotiating for time alone
- Tears
- Sensitivity
- Speaking your truth

Negotiating for Time Alone

> "I finally figured out that if I put it on my calendar ahead of time and didn't stuff my schedule full, then I was prepared. And I wondered, 'Why did I have to wait 'til I was 35 to realize this?'"
> ~Kim, Health Care Practitioner.

You may feel much less social when you are pre-menstrual, or during your period. However, you can learn to anticipate that feeling, so it won't surprise you every time, and you can help the people around you to plan for it, too.

Have an on-going conversation with family members, for example, about the fact that you have a rhythmic need for time to yourself. Explain how they can help this go smoothly for you by saying or doing certain things (and not saying or doing other things...). It does not need to be a big surprise, or viewed as a problem. It's just the "season" you're in.

When you are actually feeling the desire for time alone is not the time to be explaining yourself (and most likely getting into an exhausting argument)!

Many women realize, after the fact, that they effectively got some space for themselves by stomping off and slamming the door behind them! Tempers can be short when you are at this phase of your month, and it may just be a big signal that what you really want is some time out. Time to just de-compress, do nothing, do something creative, go for a walk, and just be un-interrupted for awhile. No need to explain yourself or how you feel to anyone.

Trying to explain yourself at this time can be very aggravating, because your energy is in a more dreamlike or intuitive state, and very inwardly-focused. This is highly valuable and potent energy, but it needs space. It *cannot* explain itself in any logical way. It is meant to be cultivated within you and expressed as Truth when you are ready.

Negotiate this with the appropriate people ahead of time. Then, when the time comes, just claim the need. "I need some time for myself. I don't want to be interrupted for awhile. I will need to talk to you later." The way to avoid an argument, if necessary, is to realize that the other person does not have to understand or agree with you. You do not need to discuss it or explain yourself, at that moment.

Just take a deep breath, take your time out, and talk about it later. This way, you are conserving valuable energy and taking care of yourself.

I'd love to hear your suggestions and ideas after you've experimented with how to make this work for you! You can find contact information on my web site www.womenswaymooncycles.com.

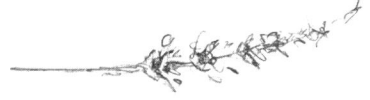

Tears

Allow tears, even encourage them.

Tears are a release, sometimes an outlet for things that have no words. It may be something from long ago that has percolated to the surface for release, or it may be discomfort from something that impressed you from the outer world – something you saw on TV the previous week, for example. One woman regularly encourages tears as her period approaches, knowing it is a good time for release, and that she will feel so much better afterward.

> One year, when my pet rabbit, Gracie, died, I cried every day for awhile. The tears finally stopped, but I did not feel done with grieving. I realized I would probably cry again when my period came around, and sure enough, I did. I welcomed the tears, and was able to continue releasing my feelings in that way. For awhile, then, I cried every month around the time of my period, and I looked forward to that time, knowing I would catch up with my deeper feelings…that they would have a place to be felt and not forgotten. ~BH

"I see tears as information, either that something needs to be addressed or a clue to something that is positive in one's life…before I am even aware or can articulate a feeling, the tears appear…I don't have ulcers and I appear younger than my years…perhaps there is a value in tears."
~Ayn Fox, "Cry Baby," from Lee Glickstein's *Relational Presence Journal*.

> Do you have a list of "tearjerker" movies you can call up when you need a good cry? Look up "tearjerker movies" online and you will find several "TopTen" or "Top 100" lists. Some of the favorites are *Beaches, Titanic, The Hours, Forrest Gump,* and *The Notebook,* also animal stories such as *Old Yeller* or *Hachiko: A Dog's Story*. Music, of course, can also get the tears flowing, and even animated movies like *Dumbo*...I remember crying over this movie when I was four years old. ~BH

Sensitivity

You can help yourself a great deal by monitoring your environment and looking for good ways to express your heightened attention to things. Really, this is a gift.

As your energy turns inward and your inner sensitivities expand, it becomes a powerful time for inspiration and intuition. By the same token, you are more sensitive to things that, on other days, might not annoy you so much, but on these days they do! That's okay. It doesn't mean there is anything wrong with you. Your focus and needs are just in a different place. So...

- Stay away from annoying things and people as much as you can!
- Limit your exposure to noise, arguments, and chaotic busy-ness.
- This is not the time to negotiate, or get into big discussions that don't feel good.
- Try not to get into situations where you feel pressured to explain yourself. Tell them you'll get back to them later. And later, you may be able to share your new view of cycle with those around you so they will understand the simple flow of the seasons in your life.

- This is more a time for imagination, "being" rather than "doing," "dreaming" rather than "explaining," and trying new ways rather than the regular, predictable way.

- Limit your exposure to violent or disturbing imagery in the media! Since you are especially receptive during this time, take a break from the onslaught of images and news. Don't just passively take them in; close your eyes whenever you want or leave the room. We can become numb to the effect of visual images and disturbing news, which impact us deeply and are hard to erase once we have been exposed to them. In fact, try treating yourself to some totally media-free days if you can.

- Expose yourself to nourishing imagery that you want to invite into your inner space. Traditionally, it was believed that what you take in now is what will fuel and nourish you for the coming month. So pay attention and give yourself the gift of lots of yummy input that will make you feel wonderful. Won't it be fun to share that feeling with others, all month long? Imagine the possibilities!

What is this time like for you? How can you create some space for yourself that feels freeing and nourishing?

> "It has taken me years to realize the importance of taking my 1st 'moon' day off if at all possible. I stay away from 'trying' to be productive or having any intense communication. It's a day to go 'in' and nurture the body. It's a day of honoring this very powerful time for a woman. I like to take a hot bath with candles, cook or read, nap and basically lounge around. I also do my best to let everything flow using pads rather than tampons. Letting go of the Human Doing and allowing the Human Being that we are."
> ~Mary Elliott, wellness advocate & body worker, Santa Barbara, CA.

Here is an Intuition Activity for drawing out your deepest knowing, and taking advantage of this sensitive time. (This is inspired by an activity from *The Woman's Belly Book*, by Lisa Sarasohn. Many more creative activities can be found there.)

Once you have gathered colored pens and paper, sit quietly and allow your attention to rest in your body's center, below the navel.

Allow your belly to move in and out with your breath. Feel the gentle rhythm. Placing your hands on your belly may help with this.

Once you are relaxed into this gentle rhythm, you will do some "spontaneous drawing" that allows your body to speak onto the paper, without any plan. It doesn't need to look like anything, or have any reason for being there. It is a simple expression of your belly—maybe just like "hello." It will be interesting to see what your belly has to say to you.

To do this, allow your arm and hand to be an extension of your belly. Let your hand choose a color, and begin to draw freely. Maintain your awareness in your belly as you do this, so you are focused on your belly instead of your hand.

Add as many colors or shapes as you feel like. Then, when you feel finished, see if there are any words or phrases that come to mind. They don't have to make sense. You can add these to the page itself, or to the back of the page.

If you want to keep going, you may use more than one page. When you are done, sit and regard your work and see what message or feeling is associated with it.

You may write about this if you want...or even do more art with this new information!

Be sure to date your pieces, and keep them in a special place.

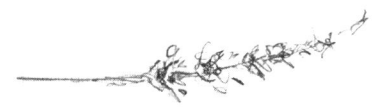

Speaking Your Truth

You do not always have to be reasonable, accountable to other people, pleasant, or available. Sometimes you may need to be the opposite of that.

This is what Clarissa Pinkola Estes is talking about in *Women Who Run With the Wolves*. In her view, we are way too civilized for our own good. There is a time to be wild...and that urge can come surging up during the end of our cycle. It is a primal energy! It gets us back in touch with our bodies, our roots, our deep knowing, our Source. It is vital, powerfully imaginative and creative. It does not enjoy small talk, explaining things, schedules, constraints. It tells the truth – so watch out!

This does not (necessarily) mean that you need to run away from home, stop showing up for work, tell people to go take a hike, or re-arrange your entire life today. What it does mean is that by taking your pre-menstrual feelings more seriously, you can learn more about the messages they really have for you.

Write in a journal at these times. Enlist the help of friends and family so you can take time out to hear your inner voice. **Pay attention to spontaneous ideas and look for kernels of truth in even the most outrageous ones.** For example, maybe instead of running away, you need to just RUN! If you find yourself yelling, maybe your voice wants to be heard. Get outdoors more, where there is green life to look at. Move your arms! Paint a big window with soap suds. Move your hips! Belly dance, squat, get down on the floor more often. Have adventures. Carve out some time to get creative and messy, and see where these paths will take you.

Indulge your Wild Woman with:

- Spontaneous movement;
- Finger painting;
- Laughing out loud;
- Letting anger out – throw something – shred a phone book;
- Playing spontaneously;
- Sleeping on a big red towel without a pad or tampon – who says you can't?
- Having orgasms! (Seriously, they've been known to relieve cramps and backaches. Women's capacity for pleasure is truly unlimited.)

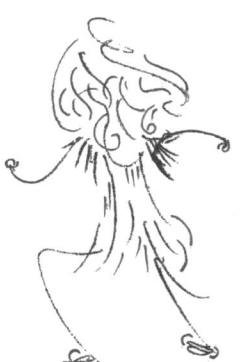

For some encouragement in the pleasure department, Mama Gena's School of Womanly Arts (mamagenas.com) or Ellen Eatough's work on Sacred Sexuality (extatica.com) offer transforming, compassionate and fun guidance! Both women have made it their life's work to encourage women to "own" their capacity for pleasure…and watch their lives become all the better for it.

The time before and during menstruation is a time of power. As your focus turns inward once a month, it becomes harder to ignore the things that matter most to you. If there is something you've been suppressing during your time of focus on others, it becomes more difficult to ignore.

> Who says it is important to have the same energy level every day, the same needs all the time? This is not how nature works.

It is a time of telling your truth. As you become more skilled at this, you will learn how to say what you are feeling while also respecting those around you. **Sometimes you may just need to be honest with yourself.** This can be a huge step. You can save big discussions with other people until a later time; for now you may just want to withdraw a little, or talk to those who can really hear and support you.

The key is to anticipate your need to take time out so you can just stomp, throw things, do nothing, be big, be wild, say what you really think, talk nonsense, be totally inconsistent, or just simply talk to no one for awhile. Lie on the floor and laugh like a fool without anyone asking you what you are doing that for. Just get it all out.

When you give yourself the gift of anticipating your needs; when you know you will have a special basket to bring out; when you know you will get time alone; when you know you will be having your special tea, or adding that extra touch to your bath…or… whatever you choose…some pre-menstrual anxiety may well dissipate on its own.

You can still go about your life, doing the things you have to do, only being *conscious*. Do this your own way. There are many ways to re-connect with your cycle and pay attention to your desires as well as your discomforts. Paying attention to these can have ripple effects into all areas of your health, your self–image, and your sense of meaning and connection to your Source.

- What appeals to YOU?
- Where do you feel out of balance?
- What needs your attention now?
- What would be most fulfilling?

Cultivating your inner life affects your hormones just as much as taking care of your body does. Hormones don't just cause stress – they also *react* to stress. They don't just produce moods, they respond – exquisitely, constantly – to the input they get from their environment, which is YOU, as well as the world around you.

In other words…each thought creates its own unique chemical inside you…and chemicals create hormones.

Other things, of course, are equally important to your health and hormones, such as exercise and nutrition. We will look at those in the next chapter.

Speaking Your Truth also has a deeper dimension, because things can come up from the past as well as the present. Past traumas and concerns most likely still live in your body and mind, and can sometimes trigger you to react way out of proportion to current circumstances. I'm sure we are all familiar with this feeling!

Yet although these feelings can seem overwhelming, they also offer an opportunity for deep healing. There are simple ways to shift and move out of overwhelm into a clearer, lighter space.

In *The Power of NOW*, Eckhart Tolle speaks of the "pain body" – emotional pain that you carry not only from your own past, but also even from your ancestors. Conscious attention is what allows it to dissolve. Simply being aware of your own feelings and reactions with compassion helps them become less automatic. You are learning to be the observer instead of allowing the feeling to take you over. Just noticing and naming your feelings or your physical discomforts will "move the energy" out of a stuck place, and begin to open up new possibilities for you.**

**Author's note: There are many simple creative activities that can help this process, which I use with my clients in my Women's Way Program and private sessions.

Don't tell yourself a story about it. Don't blame anyone. In other words, feel the anger, (or feel the body sensation of the anger, e.g. the knot in your stomach), but do not say to yourself, "I feel this way because this happened or because someone did _____ to me." Just feel the sensation itself. Observe it, say hello to it, breathe, and let it be. You don't need to fix it or figure out where it came from.

This is a profound act of self-awareness. Change will begin to happen on its own as you begin to develop your ability to do this simple practice of self-awareness.

Eckhart Tolle says that **in women, the pain body awakens when menstruation approaches**; but that rather than being taken over by it, we can use this powerful time to become more fully conscious: "Use it for enlightenment instead. Transmute it into consciousness. One of the best times for this is during the menses. I believe that, in the years to come, many women will enter the fully conscious state at this time."***

***Author's note: Several pages of *The Power of NOW* are dedicated to this topic. I highly recommend that you read through them yourself. I had a very hard time deciding what to include from the book, here, because it was all so good! See pages 29–35 and 136–143.

The following quotes from inspiring women remind us how easy and fun it can be to just let our bodies be childlike and free. It's fun, it feels great, and it doesn't cost anything! As our cycles draw us inward, we are forced to pay attention to our bodies. And here is a great way to relieve stress…something we could do every day, in fact. First, Ronelle Wood, Myofascial Release Practitioner, talks about fascia, a web of tissue throughout the body that surrounds the muscles. This tissue can get constricted.

"Did you know that your connective tissue (fascia) is not only 'connective?' It is protective as well. When it perceives danger, it contracts like a sea anemone or one of those gray 'rollie-pollies' in the garden. The purpose of the contraction is to inhibit blood flow so that if you get cut, you won't bleed too much. It will continue to contract like that even after the event, if your body doesn't have a chance to have an honest reaction. In other words, you need to go somewhere and pitch a fit! Allow your legs to kick and your arms to flail, and yell into a pillow. Because you don't get much opportunity to fight any wild animals anymore, your body doesn't physically discharge that adrenaline and metabolize it out of your system. So, even though you may have intellectually let go of the experience, your body hasn't. Find a private moment and give it a good old-fashioned temper tantrum. You will sleep like a baby. And 'goodbye' restless leg syndrome!"
~Ronelle Wood, founder of OHM (Ojai Healing Movement),
from the OHM Sanctuary newsletter.

Here, Lea Houston notes the same spontaneous self-care in animals: "Animals, from rabbits to polar bears, shake dozens of times a day to clear away the effects of trauma and stress. Your body also knows the healing power of shaking, but like most modern adults you may have learned to turn off this brilliant healing mechanism."
~Lea Houston M.A., blog: www.replenishyourself.com.

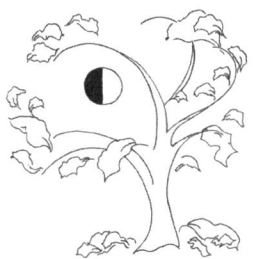

SUMMARY

Taking time for your inner life means treating your own feelings and needs as if they are important. It means taking quiet time away from distractions, so you have a chance to find out how you really feel about things. It means doing things that are fulfilling, things that have no particular purpose except that they make you happy. It means dreaming. It means listening to the quiet urges you get, that tell you when you are unhappy, or doing too much. It means listening for the wisdom that tells you how to change course when you need to.

It means connecting to your source of spirituality, your source of creativity, and developing rhythms for your month that will allow all the different aspects of you to be heard.

Imbalance can be caused by not taking care of yourself emotionally, as well as physically. Find positive ways to embrace the sensitivities and needs that you express as your menstrual time approaches. As you become more confident in this new approach, you will be able to explain it to others so they can support you. It will be easier for everyone.

Create your nest. Tie up loose ends. Complete projects, and then enjoy the sacred sense of Being, rather than Doing. Look for the expansive sense of connection that tells you that All is Well, and enjoy the gift of that moment.

ACTIVITY

1. Begin your chart and calendar. Go to http://www.womenswaymooncycles.com/calendar.html and print out a page of the calendar with the circle of moons around it. Write in the dates for this month. Now you are ready to mark the days of your last period, if you remember them. Otherwise, you are all set to record the days of your next period. Put an "x" on the days you are bleeding – or color the square in red if you want.

Congratulations: you have started keeping your calendar!

2. Begin your annual chart as well. Print out the page showing the whole year in columns. Begin to mark certain things you want to remember, using symbols that mean something to you. Decide what symbols you will use for at least five types of entries. You could list your mood, diet, and energy level on different days, as well as marking the days when menstruation occurs, and the phases of the moon, for example. You can add more symbols to the columns in coming months as you decide what else to record.

(Sources for additional calendars and charts are found in Resources Part 2 at the back of the book.)

3. Decide on one special activity that you will do when each period begins – such as taking out a special object, wearing a special "something," or going to a certain location that you love.

SAMPLE CALENDAR AND CHART PAGES:

Monthly Calendar

Below is a monthly calendar with the moon cycle encircling it, as a reminder to you that your cycle and the moon's are similar: both continually pass through different phases. You may make copies of this page at http://www.womenswaymooncycles.com/calendar.html

Write the month and dates onto your page. You will then be able to record the days of your period. Just marking these days with an "x" is a fine way to begin.

Fill out another page for the upcoming month, with the month and dates, and then draw a pencil line (or a red line) through the days you expect to be your next pre-menstrual and menstrual days.

Now, you can anticipate your needs for the month to come. Refer to this calendar as you schedule the coming month, so you know when to ease up on optional activities and stressful projects, allowing more free time for yourself as your next period approaches.

Example:

Women's Way Monthly Calendar

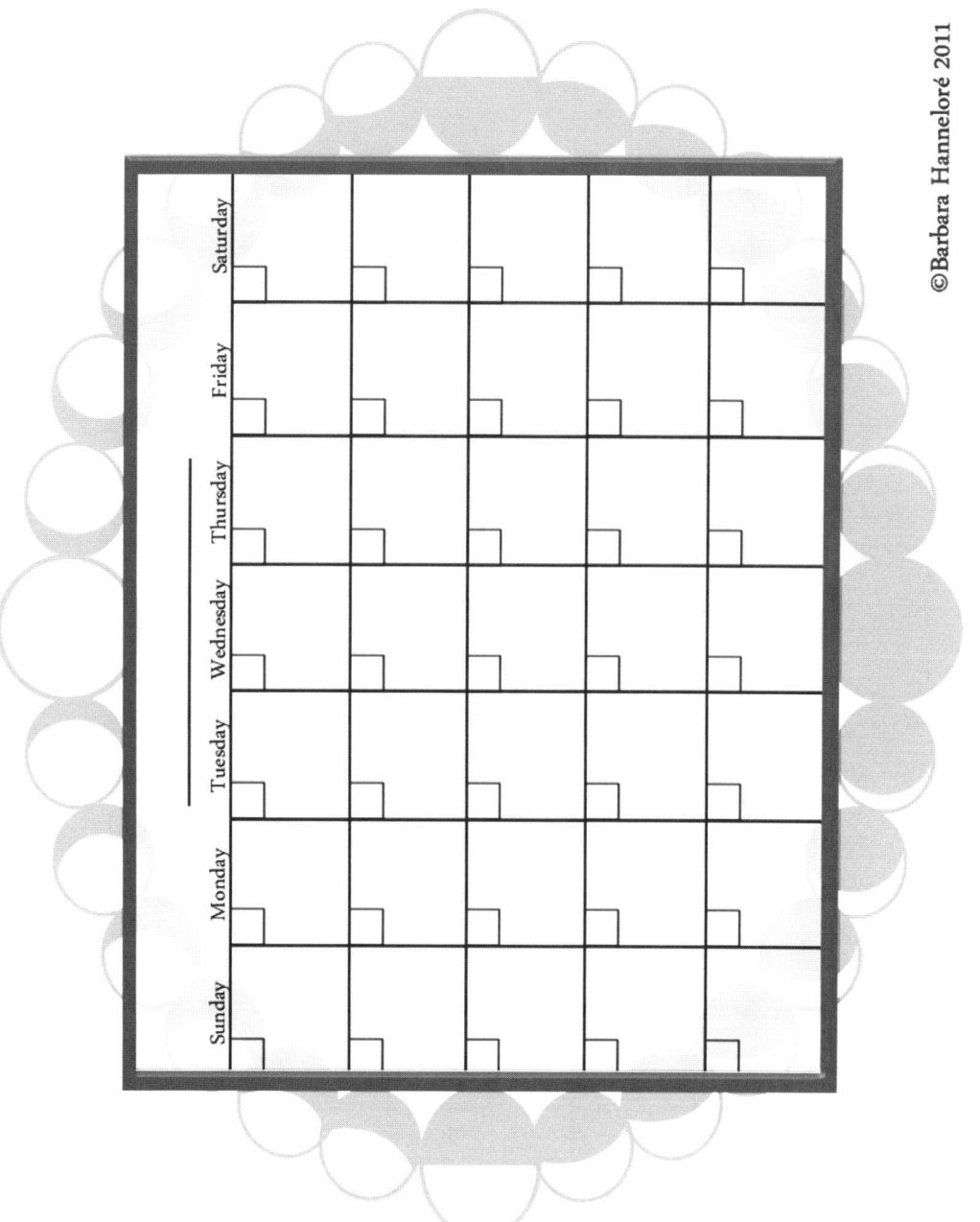

©Barbara Hannelore 2011

Annual Calendar

Below is an annual calendar, where you may record your monthly experiences and go into more depth with your observations for an entire year. Each column represents one month. You may make copies of this page at http://www.womenswaymooncycles.com/calendar.html

Use tiny symbols (either those I suggest below, or ones of your own creation) to record your days of menstruation, your time of ovulation, and your experiences at other times of the month. Each day has a space for you to record the day of your cycle and the symbol you want to include. The first day of your period is Day 1.

Sample symbols

A red dot for menstruation
A pink dot for a lighter flow
Or color the entire square either red or pink and then add another symbol on top of it:
H = heavy flow
C = cramps
B = breast tenderness
h = headache, etc.

F could be your symbol for fertile flow
OV = ovulation, if you feel it when it happens (more information on ovulation, see page 68)

Record physical symptoms and changes:

- E = energetic
- ☼ = feeling social
- mm = hungry for (as in mm...mm...good!)

Record emotional moods and changes:

- I = introspective
- A = want to be alone
- ☹ = angry
- ☹ = sad
- ♥ = feeling romantic or connected to partner
- ! = new idea!
- ≋ = creative
- ○ = full moon
- ● = dark moon
- ☽ = new moon

Seeing these symbols apply to several months next to each other will give you a visual clue to patterns that you may not notice otherwise. It is also a beautiful display of your own rhythm.

Use a loose-leaf notebook to expand on any of your observations, such as how you relate to others, and how you relate to yourself. For example:

- Being patient with yourself, saying "that's okay" to yourself, reminding yourself of things you do well or things you are grateful for;

Sample Column

Day of Month	Jan — Day of Cycle
1	HC
2	H
3	A
4	
5	
6	!
7	
8	
9	
10	
11	
12	
13	
14	
15	○
16	S
17	OV
18	
19	
20	E
21	
22	
23	
24	
25	
26	B
27	B
28	
29	I
30	
31	

- Feeling optimistic and motivated;
- Or having a lot of negative self-talk: "I'll never..." "I'm so...", and focusing on what you don't like about yourself;
- Feeling stuck or hopeless.

Notice what your new ideas and inspirations are, and say more about them. Notice what your follow-through is on those ideas.

Here, you can record:
 –dreams, what types of clothes you wear, colors you enjoy;
 –what types of things you notice, find appealing, find annoying, or dwell on.

You could record insomnia, fatigue, a craving for something, or your ability to focus.

You may notice themes and patterns over time. Some women discover a repetitive pattern to certain aches and pains, for example – even bleeding gums or foot pain – that they had not noticed before.

You may notice a rhythm to cravings for a certain type of food or activity. This may help you give yourself permission to indulge yourself, once you see that it is not "forever" but simply a desire in the moment that will give you a feeling of fulfillment, once satisfied. I used to be starving on pre-menstrual days, and sometimes felt like I was eating all day long. But I knew that at other times of the month I ate very lightly. So I was fine with following my body's desires.

I want you to have more and more reasons and opportunities to say "yes!" to yourself, to satisfy yourself and give yourself pleasure!

Explanation of ovulation and fertile flow:

Ovulation happens when one of your ovaries releases an egg. It can often be felt as a cramp or sharp twinge on one side of your lower abdomen.

While the number of days leading up to ovulation may vary considerably, the time after ovulation until your next period begins is more consistent, usually about 14 days.

This means you may not ovulate on day 14, which is the commonly held "standard" for a 28-day cycle. You could ovulate before day 14, making your cycle shorter than 28 days. You could also ovulate days or even weeks later than day 14, for various reasons, making your cycle much longer than 28 days.

Ovulation is accompanied by "fertile flow" which is a clear "stringy" mucus that will stretch into long strands. Fertile flow is the most obvious sign of ovulation. It looks similar to raw egg white. The long strands facilitate the ability of sperm cells, if they are present, to swim up into the uterus and find the egg. Fertile flow also provides nourishment for the sperm cells, and helps them live longer.

Keeping track of your cycle's signals will help you recognize the signs of ovulation and understand what is happening from week to week. This is how you gain literacy over your own body! For a fantastic in-depth tour of your reproductive cycle, go to Toni Weschler's book, *Taking Charge of Your Fertility*. For more fertility resources see page 153.

Women's Way Annual Calendar

Day of Month	Jan Day of Cycle	Feb Day of Cycle	Mar Day of Cycle	Apr Day of Cycle	May Day of Cycle	Jun Day of Cycle	Jul Day of Cycle	Aug Day of Cycle	Sep Day of Cycle	Oct Day of Cycle	Nov Day of Cycle	Dec Day of Cycle
1												
2												
3												
4												
5												
6												
7												
8												
9												
10												
11												
12												
13												
14												
15												
16												
17												
18												
19												
20												
21												
22												
23												
24												
25												
26												
27												
28												
29												
30		▓										
31		▓		▓		▓			▓		▓	

I Want to Remember:

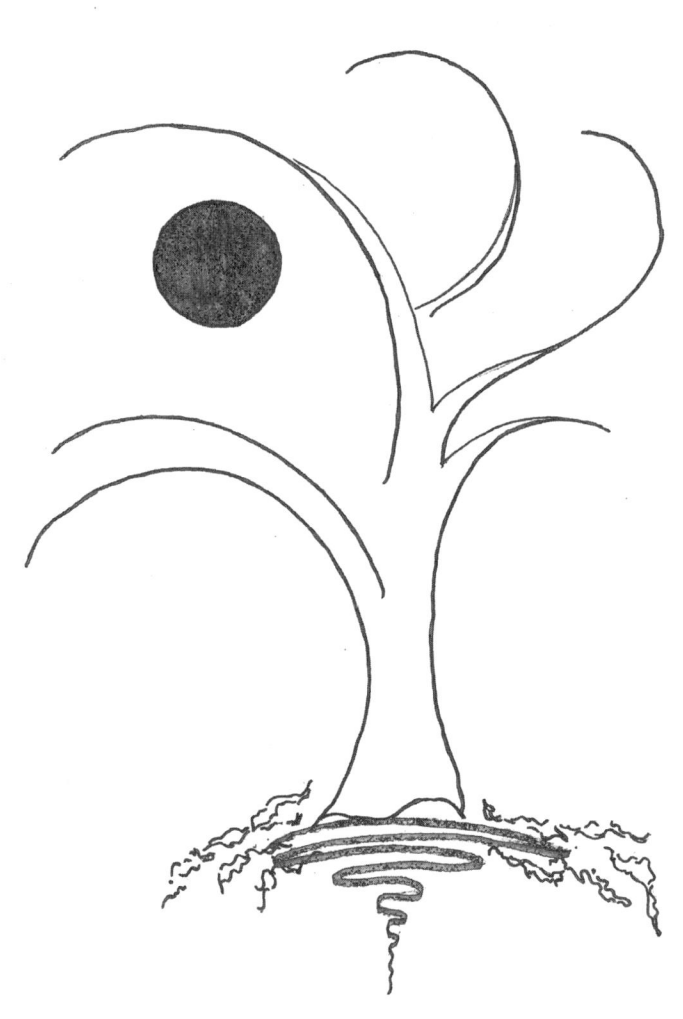

Part 3

Caring for Your Outer Life: Nourishing Your Body

Let's talk now about ways to nourish yourself physically while you are taking some of that much-needed "me-time!" You want to support your efforts to feel good on the "inside" by taking good care of your body. In this chapter, we'll consider nutritious foods, herbs, and supplements, as well as beneficial body treatments and activities.

WHAT KINDS OF FOODS ARE NOURISHING?

These days, we have so many choices of food, as well as theories about food, that deciding what to eat can be overwhelming. While there are certain things that will enhance your well being during your cycle, having really strict rules about food is not the point. It's just as important to feel good about what you eat as it is to eat "the right things." In fact, enjoying what you eat is essential in order for your food to truly nourish you.

There are many popular philosophies on nutrition that restrict or limit food groups. For example, there are low-carb diets, "paleo" diets that eliminate grains and dairy entirely, and vegan diets that use no animal products. I have friends who follow different eating plans like these, and they all seem to be doing great!

Nevertheless, I tend to favor diets that offer more balance from different food groups. (No surprise, here. You may have noticed that balance is one of my favorite concepts!)

In this section, you will find suggestions and resources that make several approaches to dietary changes for menstrual health available to you. Take this journey of discovery for yourself, and see what makes a difference for you. Your body has its own wisdom, its own balance, and its own needs.

The real secret is to find things that you like to eat. Pay attention each day to what you really want to eat. This will help you learn to trust your body about what it needs. Certain foods can be bad for one person, yet fine for another. (As you consider what changes to make in your diet, you may find that getting the help of a skilled Naturopathic Doctor will be very beneficial.)

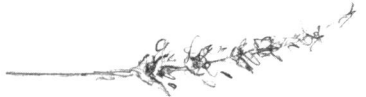

It is also important to consider the quality and source of your foods. Food is meant to nourish you! This may sound obvious; but in light of food processing, chemical additives, the cultural habit of "speed eating," and the like, it does take effort to find foods that have not been compromised or depleted in some way. So it is good to think about what we humans are really designed to eat.

Modern farming practices have altered our foods from those that our grandparents ate. These foods may look the same, but they are not. For instance, chickens that have been fed antibiotic and growth hormones, and then injected with salt water during processing, bear little resemblance to those that are raised and brought to market more naturally. Foods grown in soil that has been stressed and depleted from over-use contain only a fraction of the nutrients one ordinarily would expect them to have.

We need to step back from the rush of modern culture and the damaging shortcuts that we take with our health and our food, and move towards more sustainable foods.

Supporting your local organic growers and other purveyors of high-quality foods will benefit not only them, but you as well.

THINGS TO CONSIDER WHEN DECIDING WHAT TO EAT:

Learn to appreciate your food and the earth that it comes from.

1. Really make your food choices an aspect of wonderful self-care.

2. Eat fresh foods that are rich in color. (Colors reflect the nutrients in those foods—for example, red foods like beets and red apples have powerful antioxidants; many orange fruits and vegetables are converted to Vitamin A.)

3. Eat locally grown foods. Food grown in your local soil and season will resonate with you differently (and more healthily)

than something shipped from halfway around the world. Both color-rich foods and locally grown foods are very good things to include in your diet.

4. Look for foods that have real, whole food ingredients. Your body may be starving for nutrients that have been leached out of the soil, or processed out of the foods you eat. You may find that you feel so much better by simply nourishing your body with whole, nutrient-rich food! I generally shop at health-food stores or produce markets because I trust the integrity of their foods more. Imagine if a car was trying to operate with water in the tank instead of gas! It just wouldn't run—and it might even be damaged. So treat your body as well as you do your car, by knowing the types of "fuel" it needs.

5. Take time to prepare some of your food yourself. It's actually very calming to take your time with preparing meals. It helps the digestion. Have you heard of the "Slow Food" movement? Members get together to prepare and enjoy delicious fresh food, the old-fashioned way. It is a wonderful ritual, if done in an unhurried way. Other ideas:

- Suggestions for seasonal nourishing meals that are rich with a balance of animal products, grains, and vegetables are found in the books, *Nourishing Traditions* and *Full Moon Feast*, as well as on the website, www.westonprice.org.
- Ayurveda (meaning "the science of life") originated in India over 5,000 years ago. It is a holistic system for health that includes many types of self-care. Ayurveda uses foods as a way to balance the body and mind, creating meals to provide a balance of flavors and spices. The recommended foods change seasonally, which is appealing when you are trying to be more attuned to seasonal changes.

SPECIFIC FOODS

Whole Grains

Whole grain has been called "the staff of life" for thousands of years. Whole grain is rich in so many vitamins and minerals, including magnesium, phosphorus, selenium, and vitamins B6 and E...all valuable nutrients for women's hormonal balance. Some women have found that simply by eating high-quality whole grain breads, their PMS and cramps disappeared!

Please bear in mind that these breads are not the "whole-wheat" breads typically found at supermarkets. "Whole wheat" notwithstanding, many of those are still highly processed and contain white flour as well as wheat flour. Truly high-quality breads can be baked at home or found at local artisan bakeries or farmers' markets. Baking your own bread could become a monthly ritual you look forward to!

A Naturopath could help you make sure that you are not allergic to gluten, which is found in wheat and several other grains. Many people have a gluten intolerance, which can be mild or severe; and if they do, they find that various health conditions may clear up once the irritant of gluten is removed from their diet. That is what happened to me. I ended up eliminating gluten from my diet three years ago, after developing serious allergies; and once I did, several conditions that had been with me for many years simply went away. (Some people think that modern wheat contains much more gluten than the wheat our grandparents ate, making it harder for us to assimilate.)

Quality Protein

If you eat animal products, it is important to consider their quality. Animals concentrate the toxins they eat into their tissues, and so it is important that the animal products you eat be organic. It is even more important to eat organic animal products than it is to eat organic fruits and vegetables. Modern meats bear little resemblance to the meats of a century ago, because of all the antibiotics and pesticides they contain. One friend of mine simply began buying organic chicken rather than non-organic chicken, and watched her headaches disappear!

You can also find humane sources of meat and animal products from farmers who care about their animals and make sure they have a decent quality of life. These are often provided regionally from smaller local family farms. Ask at Farmers' Markets and natural food stores for ideas.

And as far as the value of protein goes, I received a very good piece of advice a few years ago. When I was having a metabolic imbalance, a doctor advised me to eat protein every four hours. Simple as this sounds, it had a very balancing and calming effect on my system. I was back on more of an "even keel" in no time.

Healthy Fats and Omega-3 Oils

Omega-3 and omega-6 fatty acids are "brain-critical nutrients." We need these fats, in a suggested ratio of about 3:1. The American diet is already quite high in omega-6 (found in common vegetable oils and seed oils)—the ratio is about 20:1. This imbalance leads to inflammation, which is now believed to underlie many common ailments and diseases.

Research shows that omega-3 supplementation improves mood, attention, and alertness. This type of fat, which is found in high-quality olive oil, flax oil, krill or fish oil, as well as some seafood and vegetables, delivers to your brain, nervous system, joints, and hormonal system some key nutrients that they crave.

> Saturated fats (found in meat, dairy, and coconut oil) are commonly considered to be "bad" fats. However, there are differing opinions on this. To learn about why these fats may actually be beneficial, go to www.westonprice.com, or consult the book *Nourishing Traditions* by Sally Fallon.

Since much more omega-3 oil was available in the wild plants that our ancestors ate, returning to some of those same sources of food can be a blessing to the body. (Keep this in mind for your children as well. Some learning disorders respond very well to these oils. They build and feed the brain!)

Water

Your body also needs water! Water is the agent that carries all other nutrients to where they need to go; in a way, water is the most important nutrient of all. Water also cushions your joints and removes waste. If you drink a glass every few hours, beginning with one when you get up in the morning, you'll be well-hydrated, and your body will thank you.

Your body is 50-60% water, while your brain is 77% water. "A mere 2 percent drop in body water can trigger fuzzy short-term memory, trouble with basic math, and difficulty focusing on the computer screen or on a printed page."[1] If you feel light-headed or exhausted, water may actually be what you need.

Many times, I have felt a crash of energy during the day, or just an alarming feeling of distress in my body, and one day a friend helped me to realize that I might be dehydrated. Sure enough, within about 15 minutes of drinking a full glass of water, I felt normal again. This proved to me the importance of staying hydrated. If you feel dry or fuzzy-headed, this means that you are already very dehydrated.

Even though it's "just water," you do have some choice as to the form you take it in. For example, you can experiment with cold water or room temperature water (or hot water! I often do this at restaurants). You can also drink water with an inch or two of juice or lemonade added for flavor. This is better than no water at all, and makes it much more palatable on days when water is just not appealing for some reason.

Unless you have unusually pure local water, it is probably best to consume filtered or spring water. Some water can be downright unhealthy. (Some suggested resources for this are at the back of this book.)

THINGS TO CONSIDER AVOIDING

Following are some good ideas to keep in mind, at least most of the time. Several of these things are generally not recommended for a healthy diet. If you are wanting to have an easier cycle, clearing them out of your diet is a good place to start.

Keep in mind that food is about nourishment. To ensure that what you eat will truly be nourishing, read the labels, and try to stick to fresh foods without artificial flavors, colors, or preservatives. These additives can cause various allergies and complications for many people.

- Aspartame, one of the most toxic of all food additives, is something to avoid completely. It can actually mimic the symptoms of serious conditions in the body, such as fibromyalgia, a central nervous system disorder. If you have any health problems, stop drinking diet sodas, which usually contain aspartame.

- Sodas. Actually, sodas of any kind are hard on the body. Most sodas have a long list of artificial ingredients that your body is not designed to deal with! For instance, the high-fructose corn syrup in sodas (and many other foods)—a very cheap sweetener that enters the bloodstream in a rush—is very hard on the metabolism. Even the carbonation itself leaches calcium from the bones. So respect your body by choosing to avoid these ingredients.

- Avoid foods high in salt, and foods with trans fats, such as you would find in fast-food restaurants. I never go to fast-food restaurants because I am not comfortable with the quality of their food, or the idea of mass-producing food in that way.

- Seriously consider avoiding caffeine and alcohol for awhile, to see if this helps with your symptoms. While there are some health benefits to caffeine, try avoiding it if you are having menstrual problems. Or try just cutting back, or switching to organic coffee and tea to see if that makes a difference. The same goes for alcohol (although some women find that a nice glass of red wine may relax menstrual cramps!).

- Try going without white sugar and white flour. They contain "empty calories" (no nutritional value). They actually leach nutrients from your body, and are very acidic (too much acid inflames and stresses the body). Keep in mind that refined sugar, and modern processed

> If you seek out sweets to satisfy that occasional craving, look for high-quality desserts or chocolates. There is an enormous difference between these and the more commonly found products. Organic chocolate and carefully made products are much easier on your body. Look at natural food stores and other local sources for these treats.

food in general, are very recent inventions, anyway. We are designed to eat whole foods, with all the nutrients intact.

- Many people have found relief from pre-menstrual discomfort by eliminating certain commonly eaten foods, such as meats and dairy. This is because the fats in these foods may be hard on the liver. One theory is that if the liver has to process a lot of fat in the diet, it may process female hormones incompletely, leaving too many of them floating around in the bloodstream.

At any rate, try eliminating one or two of these foods for a week or two before your period, and see what happens. You can experiment to find what works for you.

HERBS TO CONSIDER

Herbs are foods that have a higher concentration of micronutrients than is found in common vegetables. The nourishing properties of herbs are incredible. They can help you build healthy blood and bones, and regulate your hormones and energy, while avoiding the depleting aspects of stimulants such as caffeine, for example.

There are so many herbs to choose from that it can be confusing. It's wise to use caution in selecting those herbs that are right for you. It is worthwhile to learn about herbs, though, and make curling up with a warm cup of herbal tea a part of your daily routine.

Many herbs are valued for their beneficial effects on women's hormonal balance. Some herbs may be used alone, while others are usually found in blends. As with other whole foods, quality is important, so seek out sources of organic herbs when possible.

To learn much more about these herbs, and consider some for your own use, consult the books and websites of Susun Weed, Rosemary Gladstar, Karin Uphoff, Kami McBride, and others who have delved deeply into this fascinating study. You will also find some good sources in the Resource section at the back of the book.

It is important to bear in mind that herbs should be used with respect, because they are powerful! One herb may agree much better with you than another. They also can interact with other supplements and medications that you may be taking. **It is highly recommended that you consult an herbalist or naturopath before adding herbs to your diet, as well as consulting your primary medical care provider, especially if you are taking any medication.**

Following are brief descriptions of some of the most common and well-loved herbs for women's remedies and general well-being.

Nettle, Red Clover, and Raspberry

These three herbs are among those that are most commonly used for menstrual irregularities, and which can be used easily, on a daily basis. They are wonderful uterine tonics (meaning that they help your uterus feel really good!), as they are rich in vitamins and minerals. They nourish the blood, liver, and bones, and help with hormonal regularity, energy level, heart health, and adrenals. They may even inhibit the growth of cancer cells.

These herbs are "phytoestrogenic," which means that they can mimic estrogen in the body. For some women, this is very beneficial. Try one of these herbs for a month to see how it affects you, and what benefits you notice. Or alternate among them on different days, to get the full benefits of each.

Dandelion

Dandelion is very nourishing to the liver. Since the liver processes hormones, a healthy liver is essential to hormonal balance. Dandelion is calcium-rich, helps digestive upsets, and has estrogenic qualities. The roots give good, grounded energy to combat fatigue. Dandelion is a mild diuretic, which can be helpful on days when you feel bloated.

Ginger

A warming herb, ginger nourishes the entire abdominal area, and is good for digestion. Ginger compresses can be soothing to joints or achy areas.

Fresh ginger root tea is an excellent remedy for menstrual cramps. Ginger root is available in the produce department of most markets. Slice or grate a handful and simmer it in water for fifteen minutes. Add a little honey and milk to taste. Enjoy a cup or two.

Garden Sage

Garden sage is rich in calcium, magnesium, and zinc. Sage tea with honey soothes emotions, irritated nerves, and headaches. Like many other herbs, it is hormone-rich and phytoestrogenic, as well as being astringent, making it useful for easing a heavy flow.

Chamomile

Chamomile soothes and relaxes the entire system. It contains glycine, a relaxant, which can help calm menstrual cramps and nerves.

Vitex (also called Chasteberry)

This is another primary herb for balancing female hormones. It is particularly popular in Europe. Vitex works slowly. As with most herbs, it is a nourishing medicine that brings about a gradual change in body chemistry, easing mood swings, water retention and other symptoms associated with the menstrual cycle.

HERBS TO USE WITH EXTRA CARE

The herbs listed below are also commonly used and recommended, but may need to be used with even more care. The power of these plants is a great gift—when used in the right way. Be sure to consult a qualified herbalist and your doctor about your own unique situation.

Black Cohosh and Dong Quai

Black Cohosh and Dong Quai are roots that have long been considered powerful allies for women. They supply a wealth of micronutrients and balance many body systems. In many parts of the world, Dong Quai is considered to be the best women's tonic. It is rich in minerals, plant hormones, and B vitamins.

Liferoot

"Liferoot is an ally without peer for women incapacitated by chronic severe menstrual distress."[2] Liferoot is very good for the liver, and is often used as a tincture.

Motherwort

Motherwort is another favorite among herbalists for many conditions, including menstrual cramps, depression, and water retention. Motherwort is rich in calcium and trace minerals. Remember to use with care, as it can cause flooding (heavy bleeding).

Evening Primrose Oil

Rich in essential fatty acids, this oil has an anti-inflammatory effect on the body. It is highly regarded for its overall health benefits, and in the treatment of cyclic discomfort.

Evening Primrose Oil can be taken daily by many women. (For those who are estrogen sensitive, it needs to be used with caution.) Over time it may improve the health of skin, moods, joints, and more. You can see why it has become well-loved by many women!

WAYS TO PREPARE OR PURCHASE HERBS

Tea is the most common, and easiest, way to prepare herbs, but you will often hear about infusions and tinctures, as well. According to Susun Weed, "A tea is a small amount of fresh or dried herb brewed for a short time. An infusion is a large amount of dried (not fresh) herb brewed for a long time."

An **infusion** extracts more nutrients than a tincture or tea, and only stays fresh for a few days.

A **tincture** is made by steeping fresh plants in alcohol. This process takes about six weeks, but the resulting product lasts a long time.

WHERE TO FIND THESE HERBS

Several good online sources for herbs are located on pages 156 and 163.

Remember to learn more about the specific doses and precautions for these plants, and to find a knowledgeable consultant before use.

SUPPLEMENTS

It's really best to get your nutrients directly from food. Foods have a complexity and way of interacting with the body that just cannot be duplicated. This is why herbs can be such great allies, since they are foods with a very high concentration of nutrients.

There are many "key ingredients" to women's health that can easily be insufficient in our daily diets. You could boost your dosage of many nutrients listed below with either herbs or supplements – it's just that selecting an herb requires more homework than taking a supplement! So here are some of the most-recommended vitamins and minerals:

Calcium prevents muscle cramps and soothes the nervous system. Vitamins D, C, E, and zinc all aid the body in the assimilation of calcium. Calcium also requires the presence of magnesium in the body for adequate absorption. You can see why nutrient-rich foods are so important, and why a high-quality multi-vitamin might also be a good idea.

Magnesium is essential for the synthesis of proteins, carbohydrates, and fats. It helps with the assimilation of vitamins and minerals, regulates female hormones, and is a natural tranquilizer. It is one of the first supplements to be recommended for menstrual irregularities.

B vitamins, actually consisting of over twenty vitamins, are also essential to every cell in the body. They calm the nervous system and are known to help with PMS. B6 is often recommended specifically for women, but is usually best taken as part of a balanced B-complex vitamin.

Multi-vitamins can help ensure that you are getting adequate amounts of these and many other essential vitamins, minerals, and trace elements (that is, "micronutrients," or tiny doses of many additional vitamins and minerals beyond the most common ones).

Green Drinks

I found that once I added green drinks to my diet, I hardly ever got sick.

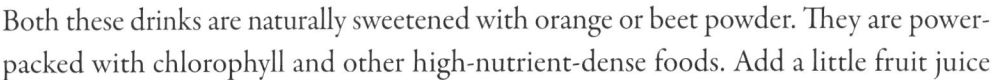

Rachael's Super Green Drink and Dr. Schulze's Superfood ("Nature's High-Octane Super Nutrition!") are my favorites because they do not have added sweeteners.

Both these drinks are naturally sweetened with orange or beet powder. They are power-packed with chlorophyll and other high-nutrient-dense foods. Add a little fruit juice and some water, or put into a smoothie, and they taste great.

Many green drinks have stevia as a sweetener, which is generally considered to be safe. However, I'd rather not eat stevia every day just in order to get my veggies! I eat plenty of sweet things as it is, without adding more.

> "A dietary approach that nourishes the body fully will also help a woman attune herself to her spiritual, intuitive side. This helps reestablish emotional flow and can often help normalize a woman's hormonal levels."
> ~Dr. Christiane Northrup, *Women's Bodies, Women's Wisdom*.

An instructor at a class I recently attended said that the one thing he recommends most, besides hydration, is chlorophyll: green leafy vegetables; "If you think you're already getting enough, try juicing some vegetables in order to get more!" He said that chlorophyll resonates at a very high vibration, accelerating the healing process within the body.

Dr. Schulze's Female Formula

This liquid tonic has helped many women find monthly balance. It supports healthy menstrual cycles with less discomfort and bloating. It calms fits of anger, anxiety, depression, and insecurity. I think highly of Dr. Schulze's products, and this formula might be great for you. Personally, however, it was too strong for my system and I was not able to take it successfully.

Progesterone

Some women who do not respond to lifestyle changes may benefit from natural progesterone (sometimes called "bio-identical hormones"). This is often helpful for women who experience severe mood swings or headaches pre-menstrually. Consult a specialist who is familiar with this approach to determine when and how to begin your use of this hormone. However, also remember that nutrient-rich herbs and a deep, self-accepting inquiry into your own life may provide the relief you seek.

AROMATHERAPY

"Dragontime" Young Living oil is a blend of calming and soothing essential oils created especially for women. It is usually applied to the lower back, abdomen, or on foot points below the ankle bones. For sources, see page 155.

Lavender has a harmonizing and balancing effect on the whole system, both physically and emotionally. Entire books have been written about lavender! Use the oil in baths, vaporizers, and for a gentle massage to the abdomen or lower back (6 drops of lavender oil in 1 tablespoon of carrier oil). The flowers can scent pillows for a healthy sleep.

> "The normal but quite dramatic reduction in hormones prior to the period is enough to cause pre-menstrual symptoms. This shouldn't be considered a disease...awareness and some lifestyle modifications can balance it out. 'Soothing' is a great word and mantra during these 10 days. Hot baths, candles, long walks...you get the picture. Sure, I'm aware that you still have to work and run your life, but plan some extra time for yourself and don't get into anything *heavy*."
> ~Dr. Richard Schulze (from his newsletter).

HEALTHY HABITS: LIGHT, MOTION, AND REST

Most of the basic, nature-inspired aspects of a balanced day have been neglected in modern life. In rural communities, the natural rhythm of life used to ensure that people got adequate amounts of full-spectrum light, sleep, and movement. Now, it is more of a challenge—but no less important. The following simple self-care practices have long been known in every corner of the world to improve and sustain health.

Full-Spectrum Light

Full-spectrum light comes from sunlight, or from lamps that are carefully designed to deliver the full range of colors and frequencies that are found in sunlight. Most indoor lighting, causing fatigue to the eyes and body, does not even come close to this full spectrum.

Full-spectrum light can help with PMS symptoms, menopause symptoms, bone mass, quality of sleep, mental clarity, and more.

Sunlight

According to the Bates Method for Better Eyesight, our eyes are solar cells that bring the information from the sun into our bodies, where it can be used to keep the energy in our bodies flowing, balanced, and strong. Sunlight travels through the eyes into the brain, and then through the spine to all organs, glands, and areas of the body.

Sunlight can be absorbed into the body by walking every morning for 20 minutes, with no sunscreen or sunglasses. (Best to do this very early in the day—after sunrise but while the sun is still low in the sky—to minimize the need for sunscreen.) This has the added benefit of setting your body clock to be properly active and awake during daylight hours, which helps you regulate proper sleep, easier weight loss, and better eating habits. More information on this fascinating topic can be found in the book, *When Your Body gets the Blues,* by Marie-Annette Brown and Jo Robinson.

Light Boxes

About 100 years ago, concurrent with the industrial revolution, much of human activity moved indoors. Since we need a certain dose of sunlight or its equivalent each day, this has had an unbalancing effect on our systems. Therefore, we are fortunate that we can bring "sunlight" indoors, through the use of full-spectrum light boxes, or lamps. The light boxes sit right on your desk and bathe you in a radiant glow while you work, rather than being designed for reading, as the lamps are. Resources on page 156.

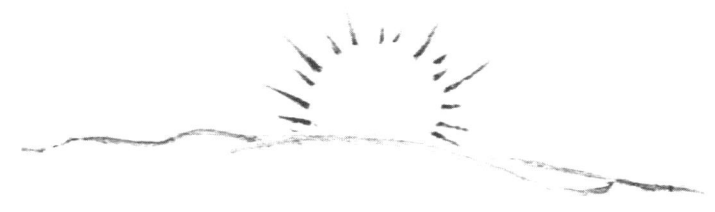

The Need for Motion (This seems to be a more friendly term than "exercise.")

It used to be easy to get enough activity just by doing daily routines. Now, however, it seems just as easy to avoid it! There are so many opportunities to take the easy way out, such as driving, using the remote, and generally having everything right at hand. Susun Weed recommends setting up your office so that you have to get up in order to go get things regularly. I guess there is such a thing as "too much efficiency."

Our bodies are made to move. They really depend on movement to stay healthy.

A sedentary body actually gives the signal to the brain that it is no longer useful, and so it begins to break down. Regular movement, throughout the month, can make a big difference in soothing cyclic discomfort. (However, too much exercise can burn so much fat that a woman's periods will become irregular or stop altogether in extreme cases. This indicates serious stress to the body.)

Qi Gong

Besides walking, Qi Gong is another soothing and energizing form of movement, similar to Tai Chi. While Tai Chi seems like a choreographed dance, the thing I like about Qi Gong is that it is rhythmic and repetitive. You do the same motion over again several times, so there is not so much to remember! I find it deeply calming and clarifying. Although Qi Gong is done while standing or even sitting, it is a powerful way to move energy, and is deeply healing to many body systems.

Lee Holden is a popular Qi Gong instructor on PBS television. He has many programs addressing health for different systems of the body, which can be easily learned. When asked which of his programs would be best for PMS, Lee replied,

"I think the best routines for PMS would be 'Qi Gong for Stress,' 'Qi Gong Flow for Beginners,' and the two newest titles – 'Qi Gong for Deep Sleep' and 'Qi Gong for More Energy.' PMS is diagnosed in a few different ways in Chinese Medicine [than in Western medicine]. But these Qi Gong routines should make a big difference."

Lee's videos can be found at www.leeholden.com. While you are there, look for the link to his "What is Qi Gong?" page, for a good overview of the benefits of this ancient art.

Yoga

Over time, yoga can transform your body, and even your life. Like Qi Gong, yoga will benefit you mentally, emotionally and spiritually as you attain more optimal health.

I feel much stronger and more flexible since beginning to do yoga regularly a year ago – and I look forward to feeling even better a year from now! Look for a gentle yoga class to get you started, and for a teacher who encourages you to listen to your body's signals each day.

SLEEP AND REST

Sufficient sleep is essential not only for the obvious benefit—full capacity when we are awake—but also for regulating weight, bone density, heart health, and more.

Before we had artificial light illuminating our nights both indoors and out, it was easier to get to sleep at night! According to Ayurveda, our bodies are linked to the 24-hour planetary circadian rhythm, and you are more fully rested when getting sleep between the hours of 10:30 pm and 6:30 am than at any other time. Establishing a regular sleep habit with this in mind is very helpful if you are trying to find a way to wake up feeling more rested.

Be sure your room is dark, as even slight light can reduce the body's production of melatonin, which is essential for a good night's rest. (This includes the small LED lights on electronic devices.) Take valuable restful breaks during the day. *The Power of Rest*, by Matthew Edlund, MD, shows you how to establish easy routines and rituals to improve sleep, and how to refresh your brain and body with rest breaks throughout the day as well. Some of these take no more than a minute! You will learn how to give your body the rhythm of activity and rest that it loves and needs.

You've probably heard that sometimes writing down your to-do list can help clear your mind before bed. But here's an interesting twist: in *Restful Sleep*, Deepak Chopra tells of a woman who realized that she had a larger to-do list, in the form of unfulfilled ambitions and desires, that was actually preventing her from falling asleep. There were things left undone, and this was troubling her! After many years of insomnia she made some changes, started realizing some of those dreams, and her sleep improved.

HEALTHY SELF-CARE: BODY TREATMENTS

Let's move on to some other practices and activities that you may enjoy…

Acupressure

> *"Daily acupressure over a period of time stimulates the endocrine system to regulate…hormones naturally."*
> ~Michael Reed Gach

Acupressure is something you can do for yourself, by applying pressure with your fingertips to different spots on your body. It follows the same meridian system as acupuncture, but it is done without needles.

Acupressure activates sensitive points throughout the body, on channels (or lines) that circulate our vital energy. This invisible force keeps everything connected and alive within us, and also keeps us connected to the many levels of information in our environment, which is our larger body.

Several pressure points on the abdomen, legs, and feet are very effective for dealing with PMS and menstrual tension. These points are easy to locate and to treat. It is best to locate them with the help of pictures; they are well-illustrated in the book, *Acupressure's Potent Points*, by Michael Reed Gach—a very user-friendly book for a wide variety of treatments.

The simple five-step exercise in this easy-to-use book also brings circulation throughout the pelvic area to relieve tension.

The PMS Self-Help Book by Dr. Susan Lark also offers simple routines that can become part of your self-care program, providing a lot of relief.

Reflexology

Reflexology treatments are usually given to the hands or feet, although there are many reflexology "points" on other parts of the body as well. Pressure is applied to these points which associate with, and affect, other areas of the body in a similar way to acupressure.

The point most often addressed for PMS is the Uterus Point, located on the inside of the foot, near the ankle bone. Claire Marie Miller, author of *Integrative Reflexology*, places the point midway along the line that runs from the ankle bone to the lower back of the heel. Other practitioners place the point farther forward, in the larger Uterus Zone that extends below the ankle bone.

Either way, the most simple treatment is to press firmly in this area with your thumb, rotating your thumb in a circle if you like, several times.

In *Reflexology: Health at Your Fingertips*, Barbara and Kevin Kunz recommend doing this treatment every day throughout the month to address PMS most effectively. (For painful periods, press the point 3 or 4 times a day until pain subsides.)

Stephanie Rick, in *The Reflexology Workout*, offers a Pre-menstrual Tension Workout, including an even more comprehensive routine of seven different points, including the adrenals and pituitary (just to remind us that everything is connected!). She recommends combining this routine with her SuperHealth Workout, and performing it twice a week throughout the month—once a day, if necessary, for specific conditions.

Refer to any of these books to locate these points. They are wonderful manuals to have on hand for many conditions.

You also may want to refer to the comprehensive classic, *Body Reflexology*, by Mildred Carter. This is another excellent book to have on hand. She guides you through giving yourself a complete foot rub for PMS, and also has a simple, nature-inspired list of "15 Ways to Relieve Stress and Tension." Visit her site at www.mcreflexology.com.

(More reflexology resources are in the back of the book, page 156.)

Ritual Baths

Ritual baths have been used for many purposes for thousands of years. One of the best known is the Mikvah, a Jewish religious ritual bath that is traditionally understood to be "cleansing" for a woman after her menses, before re-joining her husband sexually. A more modern, empowering interpretation is that this is a *passage*, allowing a woman to ritually re-enter daily life with a soothing and releasing bath that cares for her body in a timeless way.

You can prepare your own ritual bath with candles, oils, even rose petals. You have probably treated yourself to special baths before; but this bath can have the intention of deep regard for the cycle of life within you…honoring the fluid nature of the female. Your bath can soothe you during your pre-menstrual time, honoring your descent into inner space. It can also be used to provide a link to the busier days ahead, when your period nears its end. The intention you set can make it a healing way for you to pamper your body. This can become part of your monthly self-care!

If you can find a copy, the book *Spiritual Bathing* by Rosita Arvigo beautifully illustrates the many uses of bathing as a sacred act throughout the world.

Foot Scrub

Foot baths and foot scrubs increase circulation in the feet and keep them warm. This is another way to pamper yourself, calm your body, and ease menstrual difficulties! You will find three herbal foot baths and three foot scrubs in *105 Ways to Celebrate Menstruation*, by Kami McBride. Here is one:

Circulation! Foot Scrub

¼ cup Epsom Salts

¼ cup sea salt

2 tablespoons dried powdered ginger root

5 drops juniper essential oil

1. Mix ingredients together and add 1/8 cup of olive oil.

2. Mix thoroughly. Massage the salts on the feet for up to 15 minutes.

Kami suggests that you rub the feet in small circular motions. You may leave the scrub on your feet for 5-10 minutes, or longer, if you like. Sit back and feel the tension draining out of your body.

Even better: find a friend to exchange foot scrubs with. Your friend can pamper your feet and leave you with a nice cup of tea, and you can do the same for her when it's her turn.

HELP FOR CRAMPS

Many of the remedies already mentioned are very effective for cramps as well as PMS.

Remember that, just like PMS, cramps can be caused by deeper issues that need attention, as well as by physical imbalance.

Here are a few other things that may help:

Magnesium has brought relief from cramps in some cases, even when strong pain medication was not effective. Additional **Calcium** may help also.

Hot-Water Bottles, Heating Pads, etc.

Hot-water bottles or heating pads can be applied to the lower back as well as to the abdomen. This gives you the opportunity to rest, which may be what you really need.

(Some people think it is best to avoid the electrical current from heating pads, as this can be an energetic drain on your system.)

You may want to try Abdominal Packs, as well. There are hot and cold packs, ginger packs, castor oil packs, and even mustard packs. These treatments stimulate pelvic circulation, easing congestion and tension. Ginger packs, castor oil packs, and mustard packs are warming remedies that you can deeply relax and take a nap with. These treatments may not be recommended for days of heavy bleeding (castor oil packs may be too

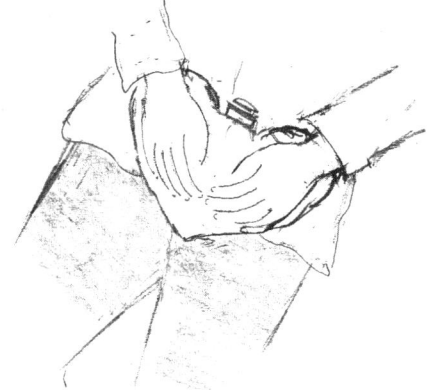

stimulating to use during menstruation) but they can be used over time to improve the health of the entire abdominal region. Check with your healthcare provider about the routine that would work best for you. Further instructions can be found in Dr. Northrup's *Women's Bodies, Women's Wisdom*, or online.

Epsom Salts

Two cups into a hot bath for 20 minutes can provide relief.

> "A gentle massage on the lower back and hips can work wonders, and also gentle Reiki can be very beneficial for bringing the body into a state of peace and balance."
> ~Emily Burger, Luna Touch Bodywork, Ojai, CA.

Abdominal Massage

An intriguing method of menstrual relief is uterine abdominal massage. This is an ancient technique, renewed for modern times by Dr. Rosita Arvigo. She studied with a Mayan elder, and now teaches this gentle method of self-care to women. Practiced on a daily basis, it guides a tipped or fallen uterus (both common conditions) back into place. This often brings relief from menstrual pain, PMS, and many other imbalances of the reproductive system.

To find a certified teacher near you, or to study with Dr. Arivgo, go to her website at www.arvigomassage.com.

ALTERNATIVE MENSTRUAL PRODUCTS

Another aspect of caring for yourself during your period is your choice of menstrual products. These vary widely in terms of convenience, quality, comfort, price and environmental impact. For some lively discussions of alternative menstrual products, and some great references to related topics, go to www.gladrags.com or www.wemoon.com.au.

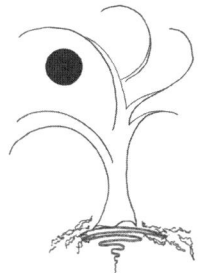

SUMMARY

Body treatments bring your attention back to yourself. In this way you can nourish your body with your own attention, which it craves! You are complex, and each way you nourish yourself will enhance you in other ways. You deserve wonderful care. Care for yourself during the "autumn and winter" seasons of your month – the "self-care seasons," – and you can have the renewed energy you need for the new month ahead.

In the next section, you will find a deeper understanding of different cultural values regarding women's experience. You may get a better understanding of how this affects your own thoughts, behaviors, and health.

ACTIVITY

Pick two nourishing things to do for your body as your next period approaches: one dietary change and one body treatment. Write them down, below, and then put them on your calendar or to-do list, and begin to anticipate including them in your daily activities.

I Want to Remember:

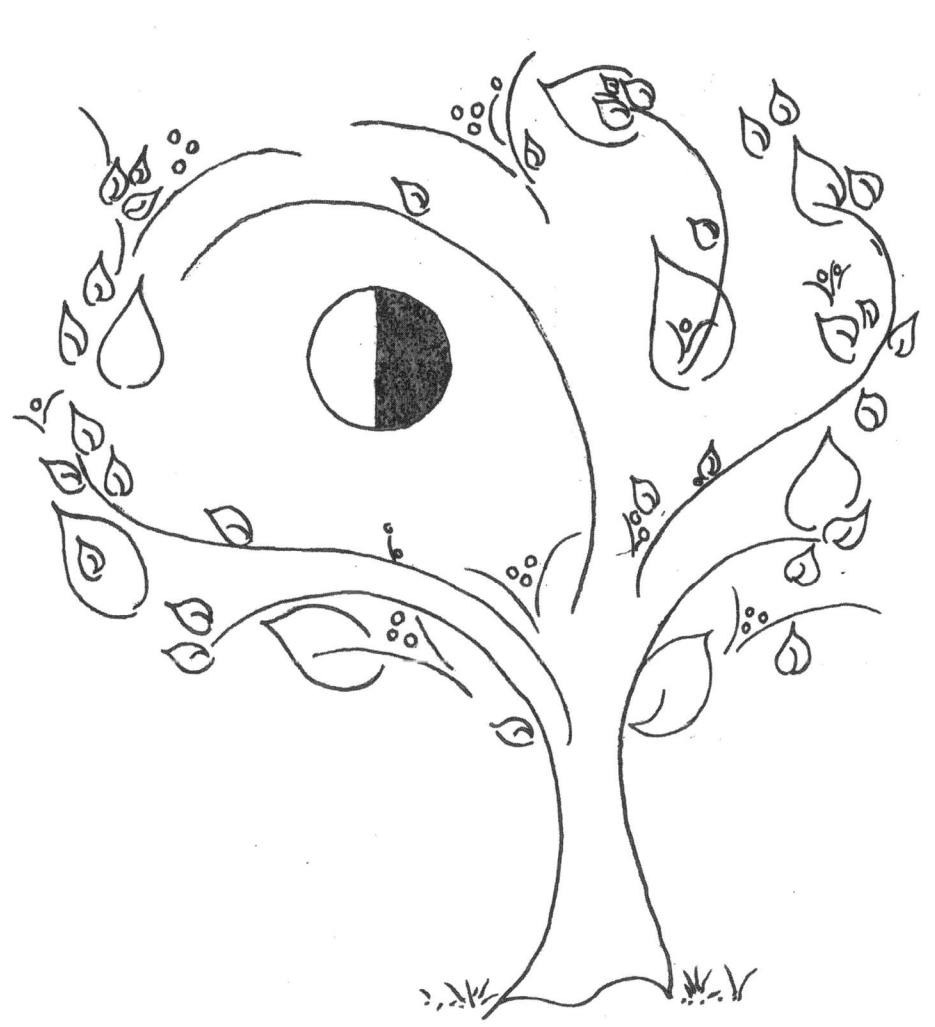

Part 4

The Big Picture: The Beliefs that Shape Cultures

The Sanskrit word for women's monthly cycle of bleeding is "rtu," which is the root of the word "ritual." This association suggests that our menstrual cycle was originally known to be at the heart of humankind's intimate, recurring relationship with the Sacred.

All of our experience happens in the larger context of the culture we live in—the messages we get from our family, our community, our nation, and the larger world.

Each culture has its own biases, strengths, and weaknesses. Some are more attuned to intuition, natural rhythms, the body, and the community as a whole, while others elevate the mind, logical thinking, and the individual.

This chapter will look at modern culture's distance from the rhythms of nature. First, however, we will look at the deeper—and older—relationship that many cultures have with natural cycles. Indigenous Elders from around the world say that our rather remarkable (and relatively recent) disconnection from the deeper, sustaining dimensions of life has caused us to lose our way.

So now that you are thoroughly nourished, pampered, and relaxed, let's step back and take a look at the beliefs that have shaped your life. These beliefs determine the type of support that you give yourself. First we'll take a look at some ancient practices, and how they can be reclaimed in our modern lives.

CULTURAL RESPECT FOR WOMEN'S CYCLES

Until a few thousand years ago, women, women's cycles, and nature were honored throughout the world.

When you go back in history to the earliest cultures, you will find that God was Female, everywhere. The female was the giver of life, the giver of food, abundant and nurturing, the keeper of the community. In this context, it seems obvious that women's cycles would have been honored as well.

In her book, *Honoring Menstruation*, author Lara Owen speaks of the "benign world view" of many traditional cultures, meaning that they "have a relationship of love and respect with their environment. This seems to be intricately related to their positive attitude to the feminine...it seems that a benign worldview is a prerequisite for a positive attitude toward one's own world—one's own body—and most specifically, toward the female body, as that is a microcosm of the larger female body, the earth."

Here are some examples of honoring women's cycles in different parts of the world:

In **Native American** communities, it was common for women to seclude themselves for a few days each month in the "women's lodge," or "Moonlodge." In fact, native women from every continent—in other words, your own ancestors!—did this. Everywhere on earth, some form of women's community was established around women's cycles;

women spent a few days of their month away from daily routines, in the company of other women, in a lodge designated especially for them.

This was the place where women would gather to reflect on the previous month in order to gain meaning and perspective, and to receive inner guidance on how to go forward. In this healing environment, a woman could notice imbalances that, if not checked, could lead to poor health, as well as catch up on her rest, creativity, and nutrition.

Maya Tuwari, an author and Ayurvedic teacher, shares the Vedic practice of women in **India**, who share certain activities throughout the month in order to keep their female energy, or shakti, strong. On the third evening of the full moon, for example, women "moonbathe," walk in the moonlight, or sit together. Other revitalizing practices are observed at new moon. Body postures, breath, diet, and devotions are all attuned to the phases of the moon. They believe that keeping shakti strong and balanced is essential to a woman's good health. Otherwise, she is much more prone to illness.

According to Sobonfu Some, who grew up in **West Africa**, the Dagara Tribe believes that the menstruating woman "carries healing energy within her and has a tremendous ability to heal and see into things. In my village, people will seek help from such a woman. They will treat her with great respect." When Sobonfu was taught this by the elder women in her tribe, she says, "This discussion opened up something infinite in me."

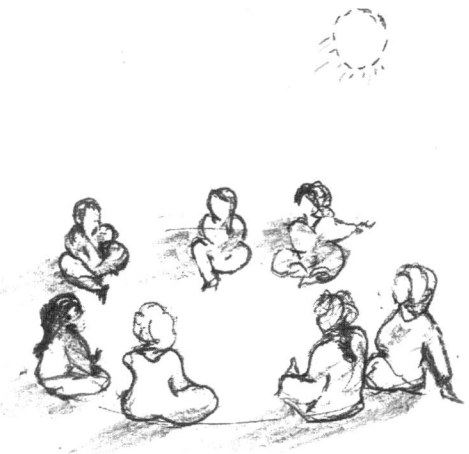

For the Dagara, understanding the value of menstruation extends to women supporting each other by doing rituals for an individual who is having her period. Sobonfu continues:

> "There is also the need for someone to contain the space for the mooning woman, as she could be channeling energies from different sources. Rituals take whatever form the woman having her period chooses. Some women will say: 'I want to be carried to this place in the village and have people sing and dance and rock me.' It's not something that is restricted. Both men and women can be involved in these rituals. She can ask them to do whatever she wants."

A dramatic account of this practice in another part of the world is described in *The Red Tent* by Anita Diamant. The title character is the tent, or women's lodge, where women gather each month—a community unto themselves— to honor the important life passages of their members, during menstruation and other events.

Brooke Medicine Eagle teaches extensively about the Native American Moonlodge in her classes, books, and recordings. She believes that women's most important gift to the Great Mother is our time of communing with Her and giving our attention to Her during our "moontime." This is our "giveaway" to the earth; the time of giving back.

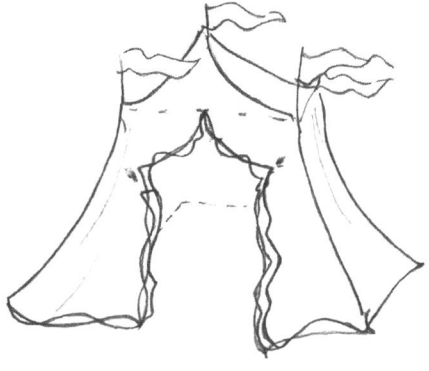

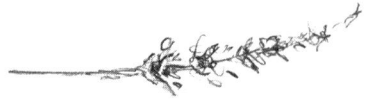

From a spiritual perspective, the menstrual time is the most receptive time of the month. Elders have even said that the menstrual time is the most receptive state that any human attains, because the veil between the visible and invisible world is the thinnest at this time. In other words, we are very open, inwardly. The world of the Divine reaches through to impress us... if we are not totally pre-occupied with other things. *This state of consciousness has power, both personally and socially. It is the most potent time to gain insight, clarity, vision and inspiration about ways to move forward into the new month.*

When women's cycles are honored, it benefits the entire community. It was common for the entire community to welcome the messages that came from the women's lodge.

Women who have learned to take time within themselves are a model of this healthy balance for others. And women who take time to dwell in the invisible world return with gifts for their families, their people. Gifts of insight. Gifts of inspiration. Gifts of caution, such as: Where are we out of balance? What do we need to do now for the health of our people?

> "Learning to relax puts you in a state of calm awareness in which you are more open to receiving helpful information and wisdom from parts of your brain that may be difficult to reach when you are busily engaged with the outside world."
> ~Martin Rossman, M.D., *The Worry Solution.*

For example, imagine if your concerns for clean water and clean air were acted upon immediately. What would that world be like?

> "Any mother, should she see something dangerous in her home, would say, "No, not in this house! No way! Not here!" And as women of the world become the strong moral force that in our collective state we are capable of being, then when dangerous elements born of unrestrained greed and aggression enter the world, it is we who should lead the cry, "No, not on this planet! No way! Not here.""
> ~Marianne Williamson, excerpted from "Feminine 2.0" essay, online.

YOUR OWN "MOON LODGE"

Imagine finding a way to take an entire day off, just for you! Well, you'd have to do it if you got really sick, wouldn't you? And life would somehow go on without you.

What if you could find a way to do it now?

Some women actually do create their own "menstrual lodge" practice, and retreat for a day or more. They arrange for friends to bring them food so they don't have to cook, just to have the experience of being with themselves during this deepest, most intuitive

> "Resting supports the female organs, so they don't get burned out in later years. Invest now, and enjoy long-term benefits from balanced female hormones. Entering menopause from a state of balance, not depletion, is the Ayurvedic approach."
> ~Kellen Brugman, Yoga Teacher and Ayurvedic Lifestyle Counselor, Santa Barbara, CA.

time, free from distractions. Most of us would not be able to do this very often, but accomplishing this even once could be life-changing.

One woman created a menstrual retreat for herself—and felt so good the rest of the month that her usual moods and fatigue were gone. Instead, she felt creative and energetic.

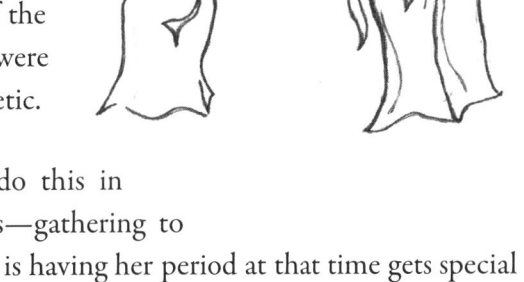

Women also are coming together to do this in groups, in Moonlodges and Red Tents—gathering to honor and witness each other. Whoever is having her period at that time gets special pampering; and whatever passages are happening in women's lives get attention, as well.

MODERN CULTURE'S DISREGARD FOR WOMEN'S CYCLES

Modern culture has totally divorced itself from natural rhythms and the concept of balance, with its bright lights shining 24 hours a day, and rewards given to people who sacrifice themselves and others in relentless pursuit of progress and personal gain.

Since menstruation is not "useful," in the practical sense, what good is it in a culture like this? It slows us down; it's messy; it can be painful and unpredictable; and modern culture jokes about it, tries to fix it, or ignores it altogether.

Our culture's values—like those of all cultures—are revealed by what is supported and rewarded. And since the natural cycles of the female body are not honored, neither are they supported in an open, honest, friendly, and respectful way.

We reward different things than earlier cultures did. We have all absorbed this acculturation since the day we were born.

You can tell a lot, for example, from the media and the messages they broadcast.

Until recently, the ads in magazines and on TV have reflected society's discomfort with the whole subject of menstruation, assuming that we'd all be better off without having to deal with it.

And indeed, modern medicine has made it possible for women to actually do away with their periods and have them much less often. This is called "menstrual suppression." Consequently, ads concerning menstruation have made a turn-around, and are more warm and friendly, advising you to "have a happy period." This is because if you still have your period, you will be buying their products: i.e., – their tampons and pads.

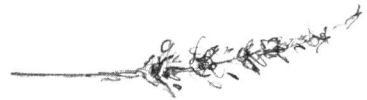

Let's take a step back from the attitudes of modern culture and consider that:

Menstrual blood is the only blood that is shed without injury. Think of that!

Without menstruation, there would be no people. Menstruation is a sign of health and fertility, signaling that all is well, and that the race will continue into the next generation.

Fortunately, you can always go back and re-claim parts of yourself by nurturing yourself with new information, more love, and acceptance. There is a place in our brain that does not discern the difference between something we've imagined and something we have actually experienced. So you can go back into your own history and re-imagine it! This will help you to feel like it actually happened that way. You will then carry both stories within you, not just one. The next section will give you some ideas and steps for this re-discovery and healing of your younger self.

GIVE YOURSELF THE WELCOME YOU DESERVE

Would you like to re-visit your own time of first menstruation, with the benefit of your grown-up perspective, and give yourself the guidance and honor that probably were not available to you then? How would that feel to you?

There are steps you can take to make this a loving and safe process now, even if you did not feel safe or supported at the time of your first menstruation. Be sure to ask for the help of a trained counselor if you desire that level of care, as you turn towards your memories with new skills and wisdom. This may be important for you, if your experiences were especially challenging.

Here are the basic steps for you, as you re-visit your own story:

1. Tell your story the way it was.
2. Tell your story the way you wish it had been.
3. Give yourself some recognition and welcome for becoming a woman.

Now let's elaborate on these, and see how you can engage in this healing process for yourself.

Yet most women in modern culture were neither welcomed nor honored at puberty. Our mothers did not have the knowledge or experience to help us, since they were not welcomed, themselves! For most of us, menstruation was treated, at best, as "just part of growing up;" and we were given pads, maybe a book, and left to ourselves.

For others, there may have been nothing. Usually this approach is from mothers who had a hard time themselves, and just can't think of a thing to say.

Let's look now at ways that we can re-consider this neglected part of our collective history, and give it the loving attention and celebration it deserves.

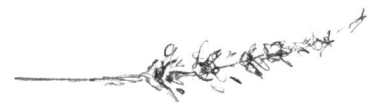

All of your former experiences influence how your periods affect you now. Even though it happened a long time ago, your own first menstruation still lives within you. It may have not gotten much attention, but it was a powerful time of passage for you, nonetheless. That day, the age that you were then, and the impressions you received are all still part of you. For most of us, this is an unhealed, unheard piece of our own story—it is something we can return to now, bringing ourselves blessings. You can connect with your "inner girl," giving her the messages and reassurance that she may be craving!

> "I am presenting a landscape of a phenomenon that exists in our culture, taking it out of the shadows and into the light."
> ~Roberta Cantow, Emmy Award-winning filmmaker, on her Trilogy *Bloodtime, Moontime, Dreamtime*, her films on the themes of coming of age and menstruation.

- Or do you feel sad, knowing you were not supported or welcomed in any way?
- Do you even remember the occasion at all?

The passage from child to young adult, the passage of puberty, is marked or honored in some way by almost every culture. The maturing person deepens in capacity for emotion, abstract thought, reproduction, creativity…becoming ready to take his or her place as an adult in their community.

The responsibility of reproduction is upon them, and this is witnessed as an important renewal for the entire community.

In the past, first menstruation was honored, just as monthly menstruation was honored. Communities had ceremonies that often lasted for days, to welcome the fertility that had blossomed into a new generation. Families gathered, gifts were given, wisdom imparted, and prayers exchanged. Sometimes there was a test of a girl's strength or endurance, or a request for her to bless the community, the crops and the animals; it was a time of power. Some societies, such as the Navajo, continue these traditions even today.

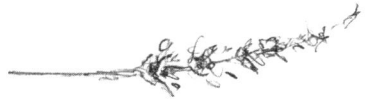

Sobonfu Some teaches that we are social creatures – and at important life passages, we need to be witnessed by our community. Otherwise, part of us just never grows up – never feels like the passage truly happened!

Part 5

Welcoming Yourself into Womanhood

"You need to claim the events in your life to make yourself yours."
~Anne-Wilson Schaef

WHAT WAS YOUR FIRST PERIOD LIKE?

A final step in your process of becoming as comfortable as possible with your cycles will be to take another look at how this all began for you. Even though it was long ago, your first period was a huge threshold for you, whether you were ready for it or not.

The way you felt at that time and the messages you received from others are still affecting you today.

- *What was your first period like?*
- *How do you feel when you consider this question?*
- Do you feel supported, reminiscent of a time of anticipation and sharing with the special people in your life?

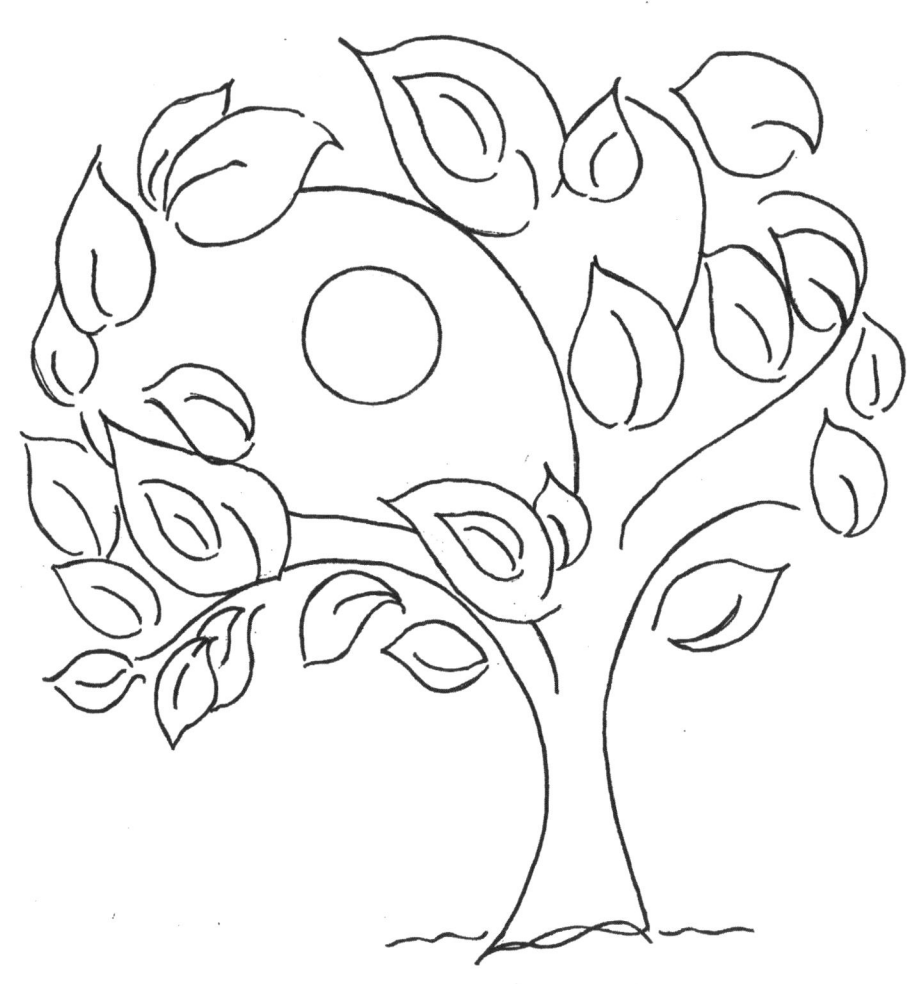

The Big Picture

I Want to Remember:

How my cycles could be if there were no shame.

How I have experienced my cycles.

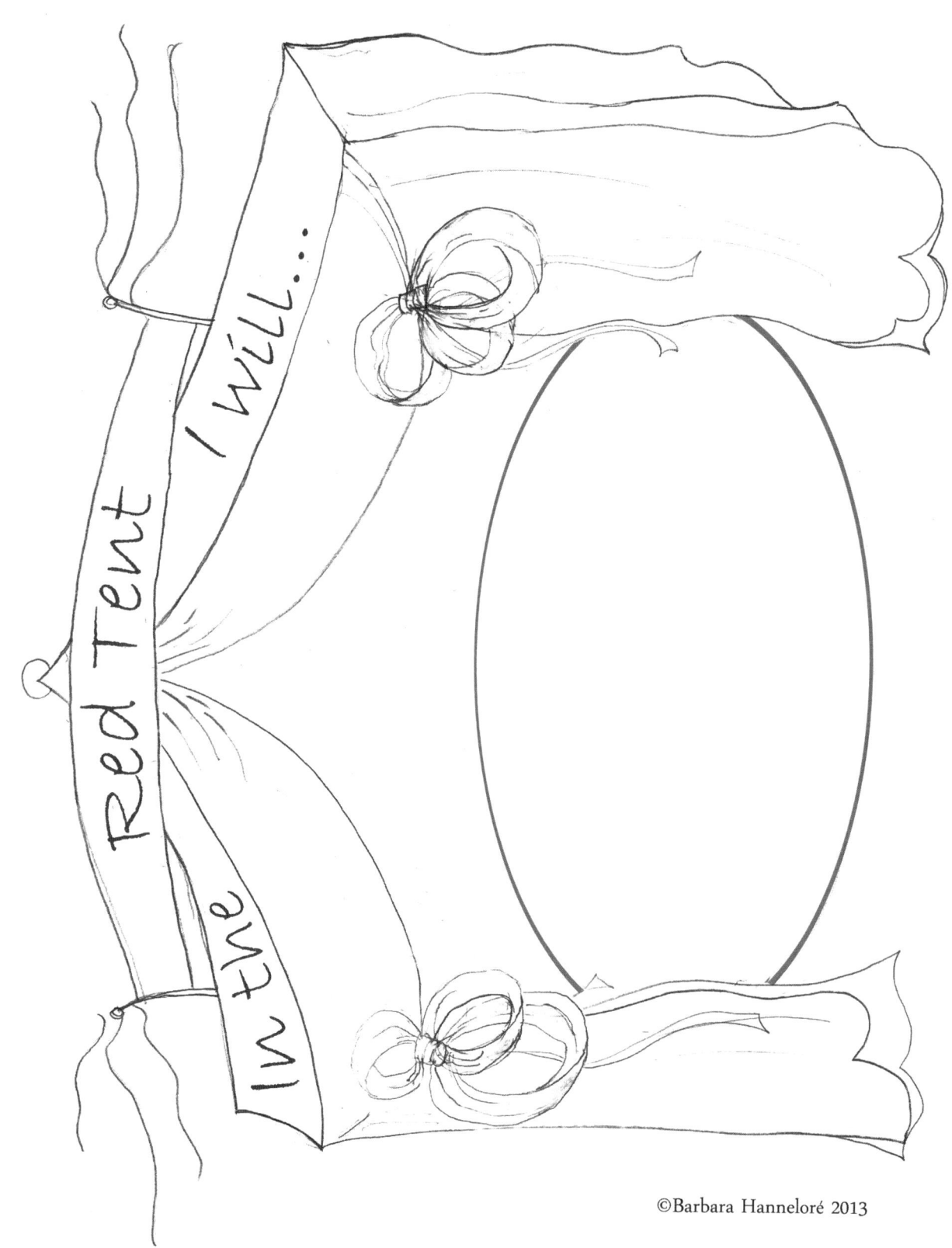

The Moon and You

Now imagine yourself in the Red Tent pictured on the opposite page. What would you do with a personal retreat every month, while others took care of your responsibilities? Fill in the page with pictures and words of your ideal experience.

Finally, fill in the two columns on page 126, considering different ways of experiencing your cycle:

"How I have experienced my cycles."

"How my cycles could be if there were no shame."

You may make copies of these pages along with the calendar pages in Part 2 at http://www.womenswaymooncycles.com/calendar.html

ACTIVITY

This is a good time to do a review and ask yourself some questions. Some of the answers may be obvious, while other questions may bring up memories or give you new perspectives to consider.

You can draw your answers, dance them, sing them, write them, or do all of the above! Record your main impressions in some way so that you can refer to them again later.

In the next chapter you can complete your review by going all the way back to your first menstruation, which affects everything that comes after. For now, consider these questions:

- What have my periods been like?
- How have I felt, physically and emotionally?
- How have I acted?
- How do I feel about my own blood? Why?
- Would I like for this to be different? How?
- How can I interpret my cycle in a way that supports me?
- What surprises me? What appeals to me?
- What do I want to do now?

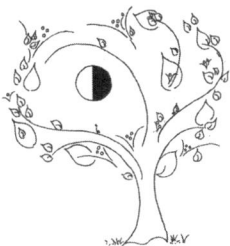

SUMMARY

Cultures that disregard women's cycles leave women feeling flawed and apologetic for something that is actually powerful and healing. Cycles are part of nature, and cultures that respect this allow women to bring deep wisdom to the people around them.

It is only recently in human history that women's experience has been devalued. We can reverse this imbalance by accepting ourselves. We can honor our own experience and define it for ourselves, and re-introduce this respect into the culture.

The re-awakening of the "Feminine Principle," the female aspect of the Sacred, is happening now – and you are helping it to happen by valuing the powerful wisdom of nature within your own body...by having respect for your own design.

When you start to feel aligned with the greater forces of nature and eternal rhythms, you will find your place in the order of things. It is grounding, reassuring and empowering.

Once I understood this concept of honoring my experience, I began to perceive the deeper value of my cycle, and to approach it differently. I began to understand what was actually happening on an energetic level every month, and I allowed myself to enjoy it instead of trying to overcome it and act as if nothing was happening.

I remember, one day, parking my car at the University and then just stopping by the trees near the car and sensing the profound connection I felt. I felt resonant. I realized that this was a gift, a personally powerful time. This was the "connected" state that people try to attain through prayer and meditation—and I had it handed to me, every month.

I began doing the things that I talked about in Part 2 of this book: leaving open space in my days, planning ahead, interpreting my feelings in a more empowering way. I allowed myself to enter the state of Being on those days as much as possible, taking time out from so much Doing. At times I was absorbed in nature, as if there were no boundary between us. I just poured myself into the beauty around me. I didn't want to squander myself in superficial activity, trying to justify myself. I welcomed the way I felt; and my experience became deeply fulfilling. ~BH

> I realized that this was a gift, a personally powerful time. This was the "connected" state that people try to attain through prayer and meditation—and I had it handed to me, every month. ~BH

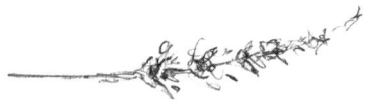

Consider this:

Who sets the terms?

Who gets to say what is important?

It's *your* experience. You are allowed to honor it. Your cycle is a part of the great Cycle of Life, playing out through you.

Menstrual blood is, in fact, evidence of health.

The Cycle of Life is operating as it should.

We are blessed, and all is well.

Don't ignore it. Don't just distract yourself all month…or all your life…and don't let this whole deeper current of consciousness go by unnoticed.

Your cycle is a model for you of letting go and beginning anew, over and over, on many levels, every month.

"In our collaboration at Cycles of Life, it has been very clear to us how much can be gained from recognizing and making space for our hormones. If you were to walk into our business meetings, you would likely be able to tell where each one of us is in our cycle! It is not uncommon for one of us to be ovulating, one pre-menstrual, and one to be menstruating. The ovulating one is usually organizing, taking notes and making the plans. The pre-menstrual one is pacing around, challenging the others' thinking process and offering the "other" point of view. The menstruating one is lying on the couch, eyes closed, every now and then delivering messages from some other realm. (These gems usually find their way into our vision statements.)"

"Can we have a business meeting lying down? Of course."

~Ashley Ross, *Cycles of Life*, a *Journal for Women*

In Ashley's example, above, the women knew where each of them were in their cycles, supported each other, found the positive aspects, and made it part of community and business life.

Just for fun, try to imagine what it would feel like if there were no shame or embarrassment surrounding the whole topic. If menstrual blood were no big deal—like a stubbed toe. If menstruation were a part of the rhythm of the whole community, every month.

If you feel shock or discomfort when you imagine these things, you can perhaps get a better sense of the cultural shame you may have absorbed without even realizing it.

There is a film out in Europe now, called *The Moon Inside You: a Secret Kept too Well*. In the preview (available online), the creator of the film says that she never understood why, considering that 25% of adult women are most likely menstruating at any given time, it goes totally unacknowledged, as if it is not happening.

Why are we so silent? Who are we trying to protect from our reality?

Can you imagine:

- Bleeding through onto your clothes, and not being embarrassed?
- Talking about your period without making it sound like a joke or a burden?
- Talking about menstruation in mixed company as if it were important or special?
- Being given "Menstrual Days Off" from work because it was a valuable use of your time?
- Seeing posters and banners announcing cycle celebrations...maybe a Menstrual Holiday?

What are some of your ideas? Write them at the end of the chapter, no matter how silly they may seem. It's very liberating to ask "what if?" and imagine things in an entirely different way!

If you go back far enough in history, again, you will see that the original practices associated with menstruation, and the original meaning of the words themselves, were positive and empowering to women – sacred, in fact.

- Menstruation was associated with timekeeping and calendars.
- Menstrual blood was used in the fields to nourish seeds as they were planted.
- Weapons were anointed with menstrual blood for power and invincibility.

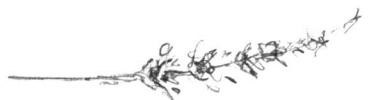

Most of us grew up in families that hid menstruation. It was never discussed; and if a woman did need to make changes to her routine because of her period, this was seen as an accommodation of weakness.

This has affected our own experience of menstruation. How could it not? Our health, our sense of feeling powerful in our bodies, our ability to really like ourselves, are all affected by the messages we receive and the messages we give ourselves.

It can be difficult to even imagine how this could be different for us, because we have received these messages from our families and the larger community for so long. But it could be entirely different, if we held other assumptions as a culture.

It's fun to consider how things could be – to stretch our imaginations as we realize that it doesn't have to be this way.

> "What is it exactly that is so shameful about a body expressing fertility?"
> Quote from an online forum at www.mum.com.

1. Tell Your Story the Way It Was

There are different ways to do this, and each has value. Here are a couple of ideas:

Have a Conversation with the Girl You Were Then

You can settle into a comfortable place and get quiet for awhile as you remember what it was like to be that young girl, meeting her period for the first time. Feel into how it was for her…what her surroundings were like, what it was like in the family, what it was like with her friends at that time of her (your) life.

And, what was the moment itself like? Who was there, or nearby? Who did she tell? How did she feel when she first saw her blood? What were her thoughts? How did her life change as a result of getting her period? Did she welcome, or even understand, those changes? Write, or draw, some of your impressions as you remember them.

> Many of our feelings and beliefs developed in us at a very young age, and are part of our Inner Child. When we were children we may have had no one to talk to, but now, as adults, we can finally offer a compassionate witness to those feelings.

One way to engage in a conversation with your Inner Girl, and make her more real and accessible for you now, is to do an Inner Child process. Years ago, I was taught that I could address my feelings as if they were coming from a child who was sitting beside me.

In other words, if I was feeling stuck, scared, or angry, and wasn't sure what to "do" with the feeling, I could engage the feeling in conversation. This helped me to pay attention and have compassion for myself. It made it more difficult to just ignore the feeling, since it was being shared with me by a child who was looking for support.

What made these Inner Child conversations easier for me was realizing that I did not need to fix or even understand the feeling. This gave me great freedom. I was there to be a compassionate listener, to let the child/feeling know that she was not alone. I was there to say "I hear you. I see you. I value you."

You can do the same process in order to get in touch with the girl you were during puberty. Imagine yourself as a girl at the age you were when you began menstruating, as if she is sitting beside you. Ask this girl about her experience. Listen to whatever she says without judging. Just let her know you hear her, and you are there to witness whatever she wants to share with you. You don't have to fix it or try to make her feel better. Just let her know you hear her, that you are there.

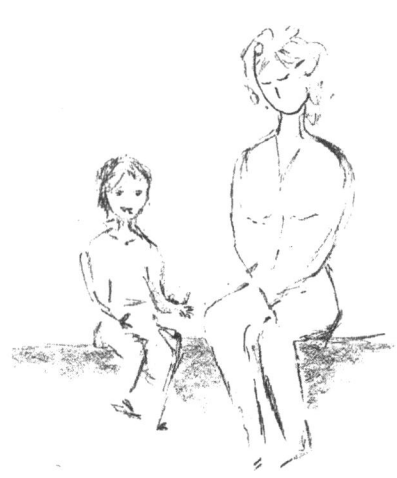

Allow this to be a tender process. Take your time. Even just making the connection will be valuable for you. Allowing feelings to be heard frees up the energy that may have been stuck within you, and is very powerful.

Do a Spontaneous Story of Your Memories

Another way to access what life was like for you at that age is just to do a spontaneous story. This may be a good way to get you started with the process of remembering.

In a spontaneous story, you simply begin speaking or writing—and just don't stop!

Carry on for a few minutes, and let the images and words pour out. If you are writing, you do not need to write complete sentences. Whatever you are saying does not even need to make sense. If you are speaking, you may want to record your words. Or you could write some of your impressions after you are done speaking.

When you are done and you review what you wrote or said, you will find that certain words or images will jump out at you, and give you a perspective or memory that is unique…different from what would have emerged had you done this another way. You can't go wrong with this technique, and you will come up with something without taking a lot of time. In other words…just give it a few minutes and see what happens!

When you are finished telling your story, allow the impressions to settle in.

You can take your time and do this in more than one "sitting."

Thank yourself for participating in this review of a special part of your life.

Hold these impressions as a valuable part of you, and then move on to the next exercise. Now you will give yourself more support, and tell your story in a new way. (This can be done at a separate time.)

2. Tell Your Story the Way You Wish It Had Been

I'm sure you can imagine many ways that your young self could have been more welcomed, more supported and honored. You now have the wisdom of many more years of experience, and you now have learned about ways that girls can be validated as they come of age.

You have spoken to your Inner Girl, or gained impressions of her, and now you can offer her a different experience—one that is the most whole, the most fun, the most safe, and right for her that you can imagine.

You can really get carried away here! Imagine family support, friends' support, and community support. You can imagine a big party. A holiday! What would help you feel most special?

You can imagine the words you wish to have spoken to you, the gifts you would like to receive, the blessings and well-wishes that those who care about you will offer you.

What do you want them to tell you about becoming a woman? What do you want them to tell you about your body and your period? Your entire monthly cycle? Your future? This is the time to help a young woman feel capable of great things. Tell her who you admire, and why. Ask her who she admires.

If possible, share part or all of this process with at least one friend, as a witness for you.

Have her be there, do this together, or tell her later about your story and what this process was like for you. You may also do this with a larger group of women who gather for this purpose.

3. Give Yourself Recognition for Becoming a Woman

Now, it is time to bless yourself with a ritual, small or large, to honor the sacred passage into fertility and womanhood that you entered, years ago. Again, you may share this ritual with at least one friend, if possible.

It could be as simple as lighting a candle, taking a walk with this intention in mind, or giving yourself a special bracelet, shawl, or symbol of power and new ability. It could be as elaborate as inviting friends for an evening gathering, or overnight retreat.

You may include:

- Candles.

- Food to share.

- Special clothes.

- Materials for simple art on big paper.

- Maybe a project such as making bracelets or wreaths to wear on your heads!

- Musical instruments.

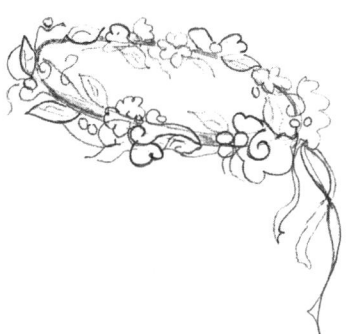

- An altar (a table set aside as Sacred Space during a ritual), with beautiful things denoting fertility, the Feminine, things that remind you of yourself as a girl, beautiful images, textures, or fruits that you enjoy.

- A song or two that welcomes you and delights in you. You could always make one up!

- A few blessing or welcoming words, denoting passage, new gifts and abilities.

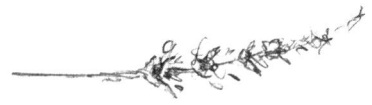

Here are three ideas for taking time with yourself as you welcome your cycle in a new way:

- **Honor Your Spirit:** Write yourself a letter, welcoming yourself into womanhood. Say what you see and admire in yourself, what you wish for yourself, and what you understand the womb to be, with your new understanding.
- **Honor Your Body:** Give yourself a special bath. Get rose petals, candles, and a big fluffy towel. Make it a visually beautiful setting. Read something beautiful to yourself while in the tub, and dry off with a rich red towel.
- **Honor Your Period Itself**: Place your hands over your belly and let them rest there. Let your belly expand as you breathe in and out. Speak kind words to it, allow it to take up space and have its cycles, as it is designed to do.

> In *Mother-Daughter Wisdom*, Dr. Christiane Northrup speaks of a mother whose intense monthly PMS was relieved after she made a conscious effort to honor the coming-of-age of her daughters in a new way. In the process, this mother developed an understanding of the damaging cultural views she had inherited, and a new love for her female body. She read, wrote about her feelings, and then celebrated her own puberty, 40 years after the fact. As a result of her inner healing, she no longer suffered from PMS each month.

SHARE A NEW TRADITION WITH YOUR DAUGHTER

Once you have cared for yourself in this way, you will have a new resource within you for addressing your daughter's coming of age. You'll be able to find the words more easily and share with her an empowered, loving, and healthy attitude toward the cycles within her.

How can you help your daughter to anticipate and welcome her cycles, and feel proud of her female body? Consider some of the things you have read in the preceding pages:

> One of the ancient meanings of Menarche, or first menstruation, is "Becoming a Queen." Girls who hear this phrase are delighted, and start to feel a sense of empowerment that is rightfully theirs.

- Seeing the cycles of nature as a model
- Learning to observe your own rhythms and anticipate your own needs
- Finding the optimal times to do things
- Listening to the messages in any symptoms of imbalance
- Doing special things for yourself when your period arrives
- Nourishing your body, all month long

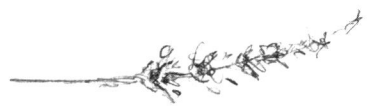

As you begin to integrate these new habits and insights, you can make them part of an on-going conversation with your daughter. Let her know that this is new to you, too, as you learn new ways of accepting and supporting yourself.

Pay attention to the way you speak of your body and your cycle. Do you demonstrate love and acceptance for yourself? Do you treat yourself the way you would treat a friend?

Research some empowering practices from other cultures with your daughter. See if your friends have any memories or experiences they can share.

Observe the moon together! Keep a chart of the moon's cycle. Observe seasonal changes, too, and how these relate to your own bodies and emotions.

Plan to celebrate her coming of age in some way that is appropriate for her. Consider her personality, and review some of the things you thought of for celebrating your own coming of age: A special gift? A gathering with friends? Music? Stories? Red cupcakes?

Write your daughter a letter of your thoughts and wishes for her, as well as some memories of your own girlhood. What did you dream about? What were your special skills or interests? Who supported you?

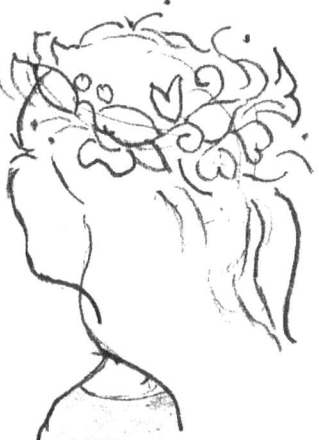

Create a beautiful centerpiece. One of my favorite things to do is create a setting of celebration in the room: an "altar" or centerpiece of abundance on a table, with so much beauty that it will be remembered forever. Include seasonal items, foods, candles, things from nature, and things that are special to your daughter or significant in her life. This can be part of a larger gathering, or just for the two of you. Prepare it as a surprise, then invite her in. Spend some time in that space, sharing gifts or wishes, doing projects, and celebrating.

Enjoy, have fun, and make this an on-going celebration of the gifts of being female!

More on this subject is available in my booklet, *How to Celebrate Your Daughter's Coming of Age,* available at www.womenswaymooncycles.com.

My own first menstruation was pretty non-eventful: my mother was helpful and encouraging, and had a box of pads ready, although she didn't have a lot to say. I remember going out to the backyard and hanging upside-down by my knees from the swing set...maybe trying to hold onto my childhood, since I was only eleven!

I was on my way to a slumber party either that night or the next, so my mom alerted the host mom, who made sure I had my own room to change in. I remember feeling special yet awkward due to all the attention; the emphasis was on hygiene, and that's as far as it went. I must have said something to the other girls about it, but I don't remember that part! We had all seen "the movie" by that time, and my mom had prepared me a bit.

I have done two events with friends, in my adult years, to honor our passage into womanhood. We gathered to share our stories (some quite difficult), create gifts for ourselves, adorn ourselves, witness each other, dance, sing and feast! We created a memory that now lives within us.

I also, now, facilitate these events for other women.
It is always a joy to behold the deep meaning that can come from even a few words and gestures, as we create a sacred, intentional space to share each others' passage. ~BH

SUMMARY

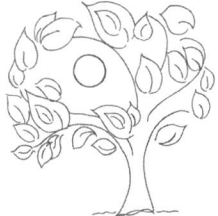

Someone once said "The Wrongs of Passage," rather than "The Rites of Passage," would be a good term for the way puberty is addressed in modern culture, the first culture that does not acknowledge this passage in some way. Silence, in itself, is a powerful message, implying that the huge change a girl experiences at first menstruation is no big deal, and even somewhat shameful. Fortunately, you can go back and re-consider your own coming of age. You can give yourself new messages and celebrate yourself, now!

The three main parts of this are: (1) to first remember your own story the way it was, then (2) to re-imagine it the way you wish it had been, and finally, (3) to give yourself the celebration you never had! It is never too late to welcome yourself into womanhood.

In modern culture, many mothers have a very difficult time knowing how to address this topic with their girls, since they received no guidance themselves when they were young. When you spend time re-imagining and healing your own first menstruation, it will nourish a place deep inside you, and you will be able to share this part of your life with your daughter in a whole new way.

You will then be able to create a strong foundation for more complete self-acceptance and health for both yourself and your daughter. Finding ways that fit her personality, you can help her learn about her cycle as the great circle that it is—containing her experience and showing her different parts of herself, week after week, and month after month.

ACTIVITY

1. Have a conversation with your Inner Girl, as if she is sitting beside you. Look at her and appreciate her.

   - Tell her that growing up is a gradual process, and it is fine for her to take her time.
   - Tell her you know she feels awkward sometimes. Say whatever you think would mean the most for her to hear.
   - What you want to do is let her know that you see her and honor her, and want to help her. You want her to hear, from you, the special things about growing up. The special things about being female, and having a cycle.
   - Tell her what you have learned about nature, and how it is reflected in her body, and in her life. How it can help her to maintain balance, stay healthy, and care for herself.
   - If you are uncomfortable with this process or it feels inauthentic to you, take some time with it...take it slow...be kind to yourself, just as you want to be kind to her! Try telling your Inner Girl three things you have learned, and how they could help her as she grows up.

2. Choose something to do for your "Inner Girl," in honor of her first period. You can give her something, make something for her, take her somewhere, sing her a song...have fun with this, just creating a special moment.

3. Tell a friend something you have learned from this process and how you think it could make a difference for you.

4. Write a letter to yourself as you were when you were a young girl.

    - Tell her your wishes for her, the strengths and talents you see in her.
    - Tell her what you have learned that you can share with her now.

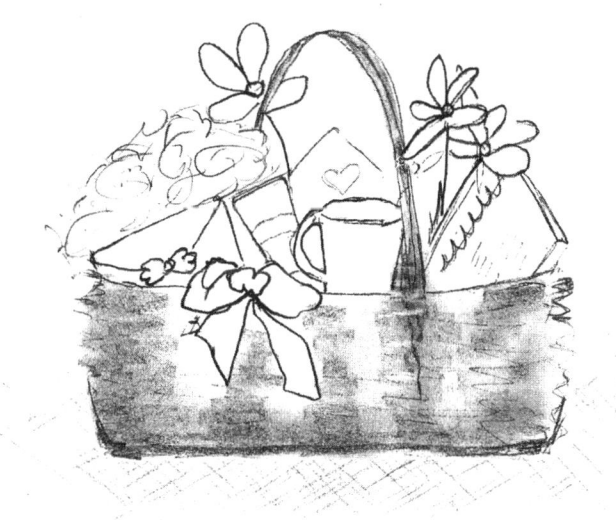

The Moon and You

I Want to Remember:

Author's Note

Throughout this book is an abundance of suggestions and activities for reclaiming the value of your menstrual cycles, with the idea that your cycles are not designed to get in your way, but rather to support and guide you.

Finding your own inner connection to the larger rhythms of life will help you feel secure in the power of resources and wisdom that are much greater than you. The *key* is interest and engagement with your own process as you create a rhythm to life that appeals to you, and discover for yourself the difference it can make.

Some of these ideas may not appeal to you at this moment, but can serve as a resource for you in the future. My intention and hope is that this book will plant seeds for nurturing you when you need, or simply wish, to take better care of yourself.

At that time, remember that your cycle can be an ally – a source of answers, creativity and insight. Just remember to find and nurture the rhythm within yourself: a guide for balance and harmony, to help you stay strong.

I'd love to hear about how this works for you! Please contact me at http://www.womenswaymooncycles.com or http://www.facebook.com/WomensWayMoonCycles to continue this conversation and learn about classes and talks that you may also enjoy.

Blessings to you, and may you find Sacred Space in daily life.

References

The tall grey clouds of evening,
The rosy mountain sky,
The breath of pause at sunset
The crows as they fly by,

The tree that frames the moonlight,
The prayer as night begins,
I stand in silent wonder
To let the Beauty in.

~Barbara Hanneloré, 2004.

References and Additional Resources

Quotes, Cover Page:
    Sarasohn, Lisa. *The Woman's Belly Book*. (19) (43)
    For full citation of any quote, see Book List that starts on page 159.

PART 1: LEARNING THE VALUE OF CYCLE

Quotes:
    Chopra, Deepak. *Restful Sleep*. (42)
    Lassiter, Judith. *Relax and Renew; restful Yoga for stressful times*. (157)
    Northrup, Dr. Christiane. *Women's Bodies, Women's Wisdom*. (109)
    Northrup, Dr. Christiane. *Women's Bodies, Women's Wisdom*. (103, 105)
    Pope, Alexandra. *The Woman's Quest*. (12)
    Pope, Alexandra. *The Woman's Quest*. (16)
    Tiwari, Maya. *The Path of Practice*. (95)
    Uphoff, Karin C. *Botanical Body Care*. (163)

PART 2: CARING FOR YOUR INNER LIFE

Quotes:
    Fox, Ayn, "Cry Baby," from Lee Glickstein's online newsletter, Relational Presence Journal, Feb 12, 2011
    Parry, Danaan. Essene *Book of Meditations and Blessings*. (36)
    Tiwari, Maya. *The Path of Practice*. (97)
    Uphoff, Karin C. *Botanical Body Care*. (36)

Other Resources:

My Moon Cards: www.mymooncards.com

Additional calendars and charts:

Cycles of Life: a Journal for Women has twelve pages, one for each month, allowing you to use the journal for a year.

www.holyhormones.com (Go to the Education page on this site for charts.)

Alisa Vitti: www.FloLiving.com

About aligning your cycle with the moon:
- Brooke Medicine Eagle, *Buffalo Woman Comes Singing,* p. 330
- Dr. Christiane Northrup, *Women's Bodies, Women's Wisdom*, p. 129

The Meaning and Value of Sabbath:
- Penelope Shuttle and Peter Redgrove, *The Wise Wound,* p. 217–222
- Judy Grahn, *Blood, Bread and Roses,* p.15
- Wayne Muller's books and tapes on Sabbath: www.waynemuller.com

For more on tears: Dianea Kohl's, *Tears are Truth, Waiting to be Spoken*

For simple creative exercises to get your feelings onto the page:
- Lucia Capaccione, *The Well Being Journal* www.expressivearts.com
- Lisa Sarasohn, *The Woman's Belly Book*

Encouragement for sensuality and pleasure:
- Ellen Eatough, www.extatica.com
- Mama Gena's School of Womanly Arts, www.mamagenas.com

Fertility awareness helps you tune in to all your monthly rhythms. Some sources for fertility awareness education:
- www.fertaware.com
- lotusfertility.com
- Justisse.com

- Katie Singer, *Honoring Our Cycles, a Natural Family Planning Book*
- Weschler, Toni, *Taking Charge of Your Fertility*

PART 3: CARING FOR YOUR OUTER LIFE

Quotes:

[1] About water: http://www.enviroalternatives.com/waterdrinking.html
[2] About Liferoot: Susun Weed, *New Menopausal Years, the Wise Woman Way*, (155)
Gach, Michael Reed. *Acupressure's Potent Points*. (167)
Northrup, Dr. Christiane. *Women's Bodies, Women's Wisdom*. (126)

Other Resources:

FOODS

Benefits of Omega oils:
- Artemis P. Simopoulos, MD, *The Omega Diet*
- Dr. Christiane Northrup, *Mother/Daughter Wisdom*
- Dr. J. Stordy, *The LCP Solution*

Healthy Fats:
- www.westonprice.com
- Sally Fallon, *Nourishing Traditions*
- Dr. Andrew Weil: www.drweil.com
- Ayurveda: www.drblossom.com "life as medicine"

Gluten intolerance or allergy:
- *Spirituality and Health Magazine*, Jan/Feb 2012, "Wheat Belly" article.

Benefits of water:
Dr. Fereydoon Batmanghelidj, www.watercure.com

Sources for bottled water:
- Arrowhead and Fiji waters both are said to have a good pH balance.

HERBS

- Susun Weed, www.susunweed.com
- Karin Uphoff, Botanical Body Care, www.karinuphoff.com
- www.mountainroseherbs.com
- Ginger Tea recipe: Michael Reed Gach, *Acupressure's Potent Points*, pp 167.

Vitex: *The Women's Herb and New Menopausal Years, the Wise Woman Way*

Evening Primrose: www.dailyglow.com/benefits-and-uses-of-evening-primrose-oil.html

Quote on Liferoot:

- Susun Weed, *New Menopausal Years, the Wise Woman Way*, pp 155.

Lavender:

- Lawless, *Lavender Oil*.
- Susun Weed, *New Menopausal Years, the Wise Woman Way*.

Dragon Time Young Living Oil: www.maryelliott.org (Go to her Aromatherapy page.)

SUPPLEMENTS

Magnesium: Stella Weller, *Pain Free Periods*, pp 50.

Green Drinks:

- Dr Schulze Superfood: www.herbdoc.com.
- Rachael's Jean's Ultimate Green Drink: www.empoweredherbals.com.
- HealthForce SuperFoods Vitamineral Green: www.healthforce.com.

Progesterone:

- Dr. Christiane Northrup, *Women's Bodies, Women's Wisdom* pp 132–134.
- Saundra McKenna C.N.M., *The Phytogenic Hormone Solution*
- Susun Weed, www.susunweed.com

HEALTHY HABITS

Full Spectrum Light:
- Bates method: www.cleareyesight.info
- Light boxes and lamps are available at www.gaiam.com, or www.ottlite.com.

Qi Gong:
- Lee Holden, www.leeholden.com.
- Jessica Kolbe, www.qigongsb.com. Jessica offers Qi Gong and Tai Chi via Skype, and has a DVD, complete with her Animal Frolics Exercises!

Reflexology:
- Claire Marie Miller, *Integrative Reflexology*. clairemariemiller.com.
- Michael Reed Gach, *Acupressure's Potent Points*. Also see www.acupressure.com for many more helpful books by the same author.
- Dr. Susan Lark, *PMS Self-Help Book*.
- Barbara and Kevin Kunz, *Reflexology: Health at Your Fingertips*.
- Stephanie Rick, *The Reflexology Workout*.
- Mildred Carter, Body Reflexology www.mcreflexology.com.

Additional reflexology and acupressure resources:
- Laura Norman, author of *Feet First*, recommends pressing the kidney, thyroid, and parathyroid points in addition to the uterus points, as these will address calcium levels, endocrine balance, and fluid retention.
- *Woman Heal Thyself*, by Jeanne Elizabeth Blum, has a routine of reflexology points specifically for women's hormonal balance.

Exercise:
- Chris Crowley, *Younger Next Year for Women*.

Cloth menstrual pads:
- www.gladrags.com or www.wemoon.com.au

PART 4: THE BIG PICTURE

Quotes:

    Owen, Lara, on benign world view, *Honoring Menstruation*. (35)
    Sarashon, Lisa, on Sanskrit word "rtu," *Woman's Belly Book*. (80)
    Ross, Ashley. *Cycles of Life; a Journal for Women*. (9)
    Rossman, Martin MD. *The Worry Solution*. (36)
    Some, Sobonfu. from *Honoring Menstruation*. (35)
    Williamson, Marianne, from "Feminine 2.0" essay, found online.

Other Resources:

Books with historical use of menstrual blood:
- Barbara Walker, *Encyclopedia of Women's Myths and Secrets*
- Judy Grahn, *Blood Bread and Roses*
- Penelope Shuttle and Peter Redgrove, *The Wise Wound*

Books with examples of women's lodges from around the world:
- Brooke Medicine Eagle, *Buffalo Woman Comes Singing*
- Lara Owen, *Honoring Menstruation*
- Shuttle and Redgrove, *The Wise Wound*
- Marija Gimbutas, *The Language of the Goddess*
- Maya Tiwari, *The Path of Practice*
- Anne Cameron, *Daughters of Copper Woman*

PART 5: WELCOMING YOURSELF INTO WOMANHOOD

Sobonfu Some, www.sobonfu.com
Reference to Dr. Christiane Northrup: *Mother/Daughter Wisdom*, p.443
Roberta Cantow, Filmmaker: www.originaldigital.net
More ideas on healing your own memories of first menstruation can be found in the six–page supplement "Telling Your Own Story" that comes with the booklet *How to Celebrate Your Daughter's Coming of Age* at www.womenswaymooncycles.com.

COMPLETE BOOK LIST

Cultural Perspectives

Estes, Clarissa Pinkola. *Women Who Run With the Wolves: Myths and Stories of the Wild Woman Archetype.* 1995, Ballantine, NY.

Medicine Eagle, Brooke. *Buffalo Woman Comes Singing.* 1991, Ballantine, NY. Powerful personal tools for spiritual growth.

Owen, Lara. *Honoring Menstruation.* 1998, Crossing Press, Freedom, CA. Also published as *Her Blood is Gold*, 2009, Archive Publishing, Great Britain.

Redgrove, Peter and Shuttle, Penelope. *The Wise Wound.* 1988, Grove Press, NY. Menstruation throughout history.

Holistic Care

Arvigo, Rosita. *Spiritual Bathing.* 2003, Celestial Arts, Berkeley, CA.

Blum, Jeanne Elizabeth. *Woman Heal Thyself.* 1995, Charles E. Tuttle Co., Inc., MA. Acupressure specifically for women's reproductive health.

Brown, Marie-Antoinette and Robinson, Jo. *When Your Body Gets the Blues.* 2002, Rodale, Emmaus, PA. Light, exercise and vitamin therapy for boosting energy, losing weight and living joyfully.

Carter, Mildred. *Body Reflexology.* 2002, Prentice Hall Press, Saddle River, NJ.

Chopra, Deepak. *Restful Sleep.* 1994, Harmony Books, NY.

Fallon, Sally. *Nourishing Traditions.* 2003, New Trends, Warsaw, IN. Well-researched guide to traditional foods, in contrast to current low-fat diets.

Gach, Michael Reed. *Acupressure's Potent Points.* 1990, Bantam Books, NY.

Hobbs, Christopher. *Vitex, the Women's Herb.* 2003, Healthy Living Publications, Summertown, TN.

Kohl, Dianea. *Tears are Truth, Waiting to be Spoken.* 1999, Chelan Publishing, WA.

Kunz, Barbara and Kevin. *Reflexology: Health at Your Fingertips.* 2003, DK Publishing, NY.

Lark, Dr. Susan. *PMS Self-Help Book.* 2001, Ten Speed Press, Berkeley, CA. Contains charts for different types of PMS.

Lassiter, Judith. *Relax and Renew; Restful Yoga for Stressful Times*. 1995, Rodmell Press, Berkeley, CA.

Lawless, Julia. *Lavender Oil*. 2001, Thorsons, Great Britain.

McBride, Kami. *105 Ways to Celebrate Menstruation*. 2004, Living Awareness Publications, CA.

McKenna, Saundra C.N.M., *The Phytogenic Hormone Solution*. 2002, Villard, NY.

Norman, Laura. *Feet First*. 1988, Simon & Schuster, NY. Reflexology.

Northrup, Dr. Christiane. *Women's Bodies, Women's Wisdom*. 2010 Bantam Books, NY. Emphasizes the mind–body connection and the wisdom of women's cycles.

Northrup, Dr. Christiane. *Mother–Daughter Wisdom*. 2005, Bantam Books, NY.

Ross, Ashley. *Cycles of Life: a Journal for Women*. 2007, Cycles of Life, Fairfax, CA. Wonderful explanation of hormonal rhythms plus monthly charts for a year.

Parry, Danaan. *Essene Book of Meditations and Blessings*. 2000, EarthStewards Network, Kalaheo, HI.

Pope, Alexandra. *The Woman's Quest*. Great Britain.
By one of the world's leading menstrual health advocates.

Rick, Stephanie. *The Reflexology Workout*. 1995, Crown, NY.

Rossman, Martin MD. *The Worry Solution*. 2010, Crown Archetype, NY.

Sarasohn, Lisa. *The Woman's Belly Book: Finding your Treasure Within*. 2006, New World Library, Novato, CA.

Simopoulos, Artemis P. MD. *The Omega Diet*. 1999, Harper Perennial, NY.
A natural diet of balanced essential fatty acids from the island of Crete.

Singer, Katie. *Honoring Our Cycles, a Natural Family Planning Book*. 2006, New Trends, Warsaw, IN.

Stordy, Dr. J. *The LCP Solution*. 2000, Ballantine, NY. About Omega–3 Fatty Acids.

Tolle, Eckhart. *The Power of Now*. 2004, New World Library, Novato, CA.
About the conscious presence within us that can dissolve the "pain body," which often becomes activated by the menstrual cycle. This is an opportunity for transformation instead of drama.

Tiwari, Maya. *The Path of Practice*. 2000, Ballantine, NY.

Tiwari, Maya. *Ayurveda: A Life of Balance.* 1994, Healing Arts Press, Rochester, VT. Maya Tiwari's books include Ayurvedic practices and recipes for keeping a woman's feminine energy, or Shakti, strong and balanced for optimal health.

Uphoff, Karin C. *Botanical Body Care*. 2007, Cypress House, Fort Bragg, CA.

Weed, Susun. *New Menopausal Years, the Wise Woman Way*. 2002, Ash Tree Publishing, NY. Includes many herbs for all stages of women's lives.

Weschler, Toni, MPH. *Taking Charge of Your Fertility*. 2006, Collins, NY.

ADDITIONAL RECOMMENDED READING

Cultural Perspectives

Bolen, Jean Shinoda. *Urgent Message From Mother: Gather the Women, Save the World*. 2008, Conari Press, Berkeley, CA.

Borysenko, Joan. *A Woman's Book of Life*. 1996, Penguin, NY.

Brizendine, Louann, M.D. *The Female Brain*. 2006, Broadway Books, NY. Excellent perspective on the complexity and wisdom of female hormones. Dr. Brizendine also authored *The Male Brain*.

Cameron, Anne. *Daughters of Copper Woman*. 2002, Harbour Publishing, British Colombia.

Duerck, Judith. *Circle of Stones*. 2004, New World Library, Novato, CA. Encourages women to honor their need for an inner life.

Gimbutas, Marija. *Language of the Goddess*. 2001, W W Norton & Co, NY. Archaeology.

Grahn, Judy. *Blood, Bread and Roses*. 1993, Beacon Press, Boston. Also Judy Grahn's article "From Sacred Blood to the Curse and Beyond" p. 265–279 in *The Politics of Women's Spirituality,* edited by Charlene Spretnak. 1982, Anchor Books, NY.

Noble, Vicki. *Shakti Woman*. 1991, Harper San Francisco, CA. Female Shamanism.

Sjoo, Monica and Mor, Barbara. *The Great Cosmic Mother: Rediscovering the Religion of the Earth*. 1987, Harper San Francisco, CA.

Walker, Barbara. *The Woman's Encyclopedia of Myths and Secrets*. 1983, Harper & Row, San Francisco, CA.

Holistic Care

Capaccione, Lucia, PhD. *The Well Being Journal.* 1989, Career Press. Creative exercises, inner child work.

Clennell, Bobby. *The Woman's Yoga Book*. 2007, Rodmell Press, Berkeley, CA. Yoga for all phases of the menstrual cycle.

Coghill, Roger. *The Healing Energies of Light.* 2000, Journey Editions, Boston.

Crowley, Chris. *Younger Next Year for Women.* 2007, Workman Publishing, NY.

Hahn, Linaya. *PMS – Solving the Puzzle.* 1995, Chicago Spectrum Press, Evanston, IL.

Trudeau, Renee. *The Mother's Guide to Self-Renewal.* 2008, Balanced Living Press, Austin, TX. Includes a resource at the end for Women's Personal Renewal Groups.

Szumowski, Laura. *Cycling: A Guide to Menstruation.* 2010, Zoo-Mouse-Key Press, MI.

Weller, Stella. *Pain Free Periods.* 1993, Thorsons, Great Britain.

RECOMMENDED RESOURCES

Herbal Wise Women

Susun Weed www.susunweed.com

Rosemary Gladstar www.sagemountain.com

Kami McBride www.livingawareness.com

Deb Soule www.avenabotanicals.com

Karin Uphoff www.karinuphoff.com

Herbs and Herbal Products

www.redmoonherbs.com Has a "natural moontime" kit.

www.mountainroseherbs.com Generous descriptions and histories of individual herbs.

www.catskillmountainherbals.com Has a wide variety of extracts and oils.

www.herbdoc.com. Richard Schulze American Botanical Pharmacy

www.empoweredherbals.com Rachael's Green Drink

MDs

Dr. Christiane Northrup: www.drnorthrup.com

Women's mood and hormone clinic, UC San Francisco, Dr. Brizendine: http://brizlab.ucsf.edu/brizlab/wmhc.html

Dr. Andrew Weil: www.drweil.com

Other Valuable Sites

Global advocacy for healthy menstruation: www.theredweb.org

Brooke Medicine Eagle: www.medicineeagle.com. (go to "CD's and Cassettes," then look for Women's Mysteries/Moontime.)

Sofia University, Women's Spirituality Program MA Degree: www.sofia.edu. An incredible opportunity for in-depth study with authors Vicki Noble, Judy Grahn, and many others.

YouTube: Hilary Talbott, *Acupressure for Women*

Rosita Arvigo, Arvigo Maya Abdominal Massage www.arvigotherapy.com

Justisse, in-depth training on women's hormonal cycle, fertility awareness education and holistic reproductive health. www.justisse.com

Katie Bowman: www.alignedandwell.com. Home of "No More Kegels," a biomechanical approach to pelvic health, pelvic alignment, incontinence, healthy joints and feet, and more.

Energy work: www.bodytalksystem.com

Lucia Capaccione: Creativity, Inner Child, Emotional Healing: www.expressivearts.com

Slow Food Movement: www.slowfood.com

Women's Personal Renewal Groups: www.reneetrudeau.com

Cloth womb kits and other Waldorf resources: www.lindaknodle.com

Barbara Hanneloré's website: www.womenswaymooncycles.com

Films: *The Moon Inside You: A Secret Kept Too Well* www.mooninsideyou.com
Things We Don't Talk About www.redtentmovie.com
Bloodtime, Moontime, Dreamtime www.originaldigital.net

Websites of my helpers from the Acknowledgements page:
> Naomi Rose@ Rose Press: www.essentialwriting.com
> Jane Schmidt www.parentcoachingnw.com
> Kellen Brugman: www.kellenbrugman.com
> Devyn Samara: www.congruensee.com

Astrology

Astrology helps you know yourself better. Even just one reading can help you know why you act the way you do, and better understand your strengths and challenges. It can help you understand times of activity and rest in your life…the best times to do things. It's about Cycles, in other words! I have found Astrology readings to be enormously informative and reassuring.

Dixie Gladstone looks at a woman's 29-year Great Moon Cycle and Progressed Soul Cycle, giving an in-depth vision of your path for years to come. She and her sister Sharon Russell have created www.feminineastrology.com, filled with inspiration and beautiful art.

Leslie Stuart has been doing Astrology readings for many years with compassion and clarity, with the added perspective of her MA in Psychotherapy. Call 805-681-9915.

Human Design

Human Design is similar to Astrology, but uses additional information to determine your chart. Human Design shows you your unique, very specific design, explains how your energy flows, and why and where it gets stuck. You will learn why you naturally have strength in certain areas, and in what areas you need to find support from others. I have found my Human Design reading to be very enlightening, in a different way than Astrology. I recommend both!

Beverly Bright www.beverlybright.com

Beth Black www.humandesignamerica.com

Tamara Slayton – an Inspiration

Tamara Slayton 1950-2003

Tamara Slayton, who worked closely with Waldorf schools on these themes for many years, brought beauty, creativity, and depth to the topic of women's cycles, and put them back where they belonged: deep in the heart of a woman's conscious experience.

When I met Tamara in Sebastopol, CA, she was teaching these concepts to women from around the country, and giving lovely celebrations for girls entering puberty.

Tamara inspired our imaginations, weaving the familiar rhythms of nature into larger celestial patterns. Her simplest conversations were threaded with pearls of wisdom.

It was always a privilege to be in her presence; her example showed me how to do this work in the world.

Tamara spoke in terms of the "Menstrual Matrix," a matrix being a vessel in which something takes form. Tamara believed that a woman's monthly cycle was the sacred space in which she developed her wisdom, having the opportunity to go inward, then outward, then inward again, in an ever-deepening spiral of understanding and self-awareness.

> *At menarche a girl meets her wisdom,*
>
> *At menstruation a woman develops her wisdom,*
>
> *At menopause a woman becomes her wisdom.*

Tamara also created brightly colored cloth wombs of felt, silk and beads to illustrate the fertility cycle. These kits and and other resources in the Waldorf tradition are available at www.lindaknodle.com.

The Red Web will soon have a page dedicated to Tamara, where you will be able to learn more about her and her exceptional work. www.theredweb.org.

About the Author

For as long as I can remember, I have been fascinated by nature, and drawn to the sacred dimensions of life. As an adult, I discovered the traditional indigenous practices that connect a woman's monthly cycle to the larger cycles of nature and the deeper places of wisdom within. This ancient, internal bond between myself, the environment, and the Sacred has inspired me ever since.

After working with Tamara Slayton, I developed the Women's Way Program – now Women's Way Moon Cycles – with workshops, speaking engagements and products, all dedicated to reclaiming the healing value of the menstrual cycle. Supporting women's connection to the natural world and its gifts seemed to pull together everything I loved – health, nature, creativity, ceremony, the Sacred, and the emerging Feminine: honoring female perspective and experience.

I am a real "process person," and love taking my time. I love creating rituals and meaningful moments for myself and others, and creating space for others to discover themselves in new ways. I think just about everything is a miracle! I've enjoyed learning about many aspects of health, creativity and human development, becoming an Expressive Arts Facilitator through the Person Centered Expressive Therapy Institute (PCETI) with Natalie Rogers, and a Holistic Wellness Coach through the Coaching programs of Linda Bark PhD, RN and Dr. Michael Arloski.

Women's Way Workshops are designed for women who want relief from PMS and a generally more delightful experience every month. Please contact me at **www.WomensWayMoonCycles.com** to explore further ways of working together.

Workshops and talks are available locally in the Santa Barbara area, occasionally in other areas, or by conference call from wherever you are!

I'd love to hear from you.

> *To know that your cycle is part of something much bigger*
> *helps you be at peace with your own body and at home in the world.*
> *You belong. You are connected to things that are eternal. ~BH*

Acknowledgements

As I pause before sending this book to the designer, I am filled with gratitude for all the women who have contributed to this project over many years, each in your own way, and to the readers who will connect with it in the future. We are, together, creating a more loving self-concept which will expand to touch the lives of many more.

Thank you to my friends, co-horts and wise women Pam Henson, Leslie Stuart and Gienne Gabriels, for the decades of insightful conversations and projects which could only happen with friends who really "get" this work. We've been through so many adventures, and you mean so much to me. Pam, you deserve an extra thanks because you've been there through dozens of rehearsals and preparations and have offered so much perceptive encouragement.

Many thanks as well to editors Naomi Rose, Kate Markham and Ela Lindsey, readers Jane Schmidt, Kellen Brugman, Emily Burger, Salima McKelvey, and Cindy Gerber, design artist Devyn Samara who created several of the activity pages, design artist Heather Wennergren, who made the cover come alive, and graphic designer Cynthia Smith who put the whole thing together. All of your enthusiastic support and insightful suggestions helped carry this book along to completion through its many revisions. I needed you to hold the vision with me, and you did – thank you all!

Linda Miramontes Gray, artist and art teacher, showed up at just the right time to encourage me to use my own sketches for the book. Thank you Linda; you gave just enough suggestions and tips, with plenty of room for imperfection and spontaneity.

And to the women of the Red Web, for your visionary activism that is changing the world. Being editor of your newsletter gave me a front-row seat to your inspired activities for several years, and gives me a strong sense of community, knowing that you, too, are out there doing this work with women everywhere.

Bless you.